Caregiver's Guide to Dementia & Alzheimer's

Real-Life Stories and Expert Guidance To Navigate the Journey Ahead From Diagnosis to Hospice Including Financial/Legal Matters & Coping with Stress & Burnout

Alison Blaire

Edited by
Randy L. Cohen

About the Author

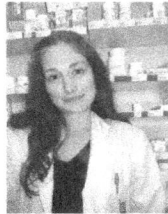

When I was a little girl, my great-grandfather lived in an assisted living facility. My family and I would visit him often, and to this very day, these memories remain deeply embedded in my mind. I vividly recall seeing other residents, sometimes looking lost and shuffling around listlessly. I specifically remember a woman screaming, "Help me, help me!" as we passed by her. I was just a kid. In my eyes, I saw sadness and confusion, and this had a profound effect on me. I couldn't get the thought that this could have been my great-grandfather out of my mind. All I wanted to do was kidnap him and take him home with us. Unfortunately, this was not possible.

Fast forward to when I was 23, my grandmother was diagnosed with dementia. My grandmother and I had a very special relationship, and I loved her so very much. At the time, she was living in her own home with a caregiver that came daily. I would visit her every weekend, and our ritual was to go to the neighborhood deli, where she would always order blintzes - her favorite. As time passed, I realized things were changing. My grandma was no longer the grandma I knew and loved. The quality of our conversations declined. She would repeat the same thing over and over and was unable to engage in any meaningful conversation. Sometimes, as I talked to her, she would randomly shout things like, "Pistachio, I love it!"

It was painful to see my grandma, whom I loved so much, looked up to, and relied on, morphing into someone I could hardly recognize. This was so difficult for me on so many levels, and emotionally, it was taking its toll. I knew enough about the disease to realize that as bad as things seemed, it would only get worse. It was then, I made the decision to educate myself to understand this disease better so that I could provide my grandmother with the love and understanding she would need, as the disease progressed.

At that time, I was an undergrad at the University of Miami, studying medicine, biology, and chemistry. As my knowledge grew, I attempted to explore the various angles of the disease, which propelled me to view this disease from behind the lens of science and medicine. Although my initial motivation to study science was rooted in my desire to help others, I became further inspired by my desire to help my grandmother.

Upon graduation, I made the decision to go to pharmacy school. I felt this would give me the additional tools and resources, allowing me to ascend to the forefront of medicine, science, and technology. Prior to graduating from pharmacy school, my grandmother's daughter, my aunt, was diagnosed with Alzheimer's, and just two years after that, my other aunt, her sister, was also diagnosed with Alzheimer's.

At that time, having already seen firsthand how dementia affected my grandmother, I witnessed my two aunts suffer the debilitating stages of this disease. This made me question if there was some magic bullet available that could help prevent, or at least slow down the effects of this disease. I was fearful for my sister, my dad, and myself, as with this disease, genetics plays a role, and clearly, it runs in our family.

I am so fortunate that my profession as a pharmacist, aligned with my passion for helping families manage the complexities of dementia. With more than a decade of experience in the field, I have, and continue to develop expertise in simplifying complicated medical issues, making them easier to understand.

My goal, when writing this book was to bring my expertise to you, my readers. I strongly believe that knowledge and support are the two most important tools in helping families navigate the world of dementia, and is especially essential for caregivers. I have dedicated this book to my grandmother with the hope of providing the necessary resources that will empower caregivers to be the best they can be and help them to be better equipped to make informed and knowledgeable decisions.

In addition to being a licensed pharmacist, I have become a professional speaker and author. I regularly contribute to several health and wellness websites, wherein, I offer helpful tips and advice to families.

My goal is to provide families with the resources they need to make their journey through dementia caregiving easier and less stressful. I want to empower caregivers with the information and tools necessary to make the best, most knowledgeable decisions, so that they can provide the best care for their loved ones.

Now you know why I have written this book. My sincere intention is that it will help you to become a capable caregiver, so that you can provide your loved one with the support, care, and treatment they need, and so deserve.

On a more personal note, I currently reside in the Bay Area with my amazing boyfriend and two adorable cats, Bax & Benny. You can check them out on Instagram at BaxandBenny. I am passionate about traveling, as seeing the world has allowed me to learn about other cultures and lifestyles. I am also a certified yoga instructor, which has afforded me the opportunity to work with people from all walks of life, including seniors and dementia patients. I have found this discipline to be extremely beneficial to those I teach, as well as to myself, on a personal level. As a dancer and yoga instructor, I have been fortunate to lead many international retreats teaching the art of yoga and dance, which I have found to be invaluable tools for relaxation and stress reduction. Recently, I have been diving into the world of holistic nutrition. It should come as no surprise that my life's journey has taken me through these connected paths, all of which align with my mission to care for the body and mind, in order to live your best life.

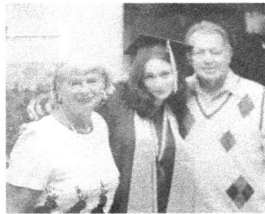

This book is dedicated to my grandma, Gussie Jacoby, one of her closest friends, Estelle Goldschein, and my aunts, Ronnie Goldnick and Fran Levine, all of whom passed away in the final stage of this disease.

I miss you with every day that passes. I hope you are looking down on me and are proud of all I have accomplished and all the things I have yet to do! I love you so much and am so grateful for all the memories we created. My grandma always said, " If you have your health, you have everything."

And in light of that, I also dedicate this book to you, for taking on this selfless journey, as a caregiver. May the memories you create with your loved one provide you abundant happiness and peace.

Table of Contents

Introduction

In 2021, there were more than 11 million dementia caregivers in the United States, alone. The story that I'm about to share with you is one out of that 11 million. It's the story of Jane, a mother and daughter from Queens, New York. Jane is a caregiver for not one but two special needs loved ones. Both her 82-year-old mother and her 40-year-old daughter have dementia. Jane told me, and I quote: "When their lives began to change, my life began to change, as well."

Jane's daughter has Down Syndrome, which is one factor that can contribute to early-onset Alzheimer's. Jane's mother, who had been living with her for more than ten years, had a recent diagnosis of dementia. While her mind was still capable enough to recall things, she was beginning to forget conversations, and taking her meds properly was becoming a great concern. Jane realized that in order to care for her mother and daughter, she would need to retire early and become a full-time caregiver.

Jane's story truly resonated with me. Having been a caregiver to my grandmother, as well as a pharmacist and writer, I felt compelled to undertake the challenge of writing this book, to provide you, the reader, with relatable stories and critical advice to assist you in your caregiving journey. Jane told me how much joy she derived as the primary caregiver for her mom and daughter. This reminded me, how I, too, considered it a privilege and derived joy from my role as caregiver for my grandmother. She said, "Taking care of my daughter and mom is actually a pleasure. I consider it a privilege, and if you can believe it, I know I am receiving way more than I give. It's a journey and every day is different."

The optimism in her story and her unwavering resolve to take care of her mother and daughter, was inspiring. It shed light on the flip side of this very trying coin. I was confident that I could convey the great purpose and need of caregiving, as I became convinced that meaningfulness and joy were amongst the many rewards, one could expect to receive as a result of providing care for your loved one with dementia. My hope, is that you, my reader, will find this book helpful in so many ways and gain insight, and with some luck, it will even give you a chuckle or two. I'd like to share one last thing that Jane shared with me, because what she shared, will ultimately tie in with almost everything we are about to explore in this book.

She said, and I quote, "I would encourage other caregivers to make time for themselves. It's hard to do, really hard! Caregivers shouldn't feel guilty, thinking that they aren't doing enough. They have to have confidence in themselves, and believe that they are doing the best they can."As this book is written with caregivers in mind, what Jane summarized tops the list of all the advice you'll find in this book. You have to take care of yourself while you provide care for your loved one. You should never feel guilty. Never believe you aren't doing enough because you're doing all you can, and you're actually DOING IT! My hope is that this book will assist you while channeling your efforts into productive strategies that will benefit you and your loved one, in this trying time.

Some of the challenges you will experience as a caregiver that are specifically addressed within the pages of this book, include caregiver burnout, psychological morbidity, isolation, physical morbidity, financial issues, wandering, incontinence, agitation, and continued communication challenges. You can also expect to learn and understand, what I believe to be most important, as you become a caregiver for your loved one with dementia:

Understanding Dementia: Explains how the disease affects the brain and changes the person.
Symptoms of Dementia: Reviews the primary symptoms of dementia and how symptoms differ depending on the various types of dementia your loved one has.
Stages of Dementia: Discusses the 7 stages of dementia, what a patient in these stages is experiencing, and what you, the primary caregiver, can expect.
Diagnosis: I did a deep dive into understanding the various procedures that are necessary for a diagnosis and the team of healthcare professionals you will need to assemble to provide the best care for your loved one.
I also provide a binder to help you prepare and keep your doctor visits and emergency paperwork organized and readily available when needed. So don't forget to click the LINK if you

are reading the ebook or scan the QR code below if you are reading in print.

Treatment and Care: Explains the different types of treatments and care available to your loved one, which include various therapies, medications, and necessary environmental modifications.

Managing and Understanding Common Behavioral Issues: Reviews the various behavioral issues your loved one will undergo and how to best manage them. These issues include sleep, wandering, anger, aggression, hallucinations, and hoarding.

At Home Care or Outside Care Facility - What's Best for You and Your Loved One: Discusses the many options available, so that you can make the best, informed, and emotionally acceptable decisions regarding the care of your loved one. I provide an in-depth view of the various types of care available, both inside and outside the home. These include home care, memory care facilities, nursing care facilities, group homes, and assisted living facilities.

Hospice: Discusses hospice care, defining what it is and the services it provides.

Support and Tips Throughout Your Journey: Provides you with tips throughout the varying stages of dementia. Including tips to support your daily routine, tips for maintaining a healthy lifestyle, tips to help you survive the grieving process, tips on how to mitigate your loved one's changes through their loss of independence, and tips for dealing with the late stages of dementia.

Strategies to Manage Communication Challenges: Discusses strategies to manage communication challenges throughout the stages of dementia.

Setting Your Home Up For Safety & Comfort: Walks you through how to transform your home into a safe, comfortable, and efficient environment and provides tips for their personal hygiene.

Managing Legalities and Financial Affairs: Financial resources and the ability to pay for care are discussed. In addition, I provide you with the necessary information to help you navigate financial affairs, legalities, insurance, and tax-related matters. In your binder, I provide an individual section to place your insurance and legal documents.

Lifestyle modifications: Encourages lifestyle modifications to slow disease progression and keep you, the caregiver, in top shape. This chapter provides you with information to illicit physical exercise and social interaction, tips on maintaining a healthy diet, ways to stimulate the mind, maintain quality sleep, manage stress, and, if possible, improve or at least maintain vascular health.

Holistic and Alternative Care: Delves into holistic and alternative care treatment options, which include different types of available therapies such as cannabis, pet, music, art, cognitive behavioral therapy, etc.

The Criticality of Self-Care for Dementia Caregivers: Emphasizes the criticality of self-care for caregivers. I reviewed the signs of caregiver stress and burnout and explore the various avenues that can help you to avoid burnout, such as emotional self-care, empowering yourself as a caregiver, and maintaining your health through regular exercise, healthy eating habits, and different forms and techniques for relaxation.

Dealing With Family: Delves into family dynamics and discusses the major challenges that you, as the primary caregiver, will face when dealing with you and your loved one's family. These include coming to terms with the diagnosis, exploring and, when necessary, resolving family conflicts.

Throughout the book, I share personal experiences, as well as those of others who have gone through similar journeys in their caregiving world.

Whether or not you are a first-time caregiver, providing care for your loved one with dementia, you will be taken to uncharted territories. Each stage of dementia (early, middle, and late) has its own learning curve, which you will probably have to adapt to on the fly. Why? Because each patient, as well as each type of dementia, is unique. While the general premise is the same, it's the specifics that you, as a caregiver, will require assistance with - as always, "the devil is in the details."

I sincerely hope that the tools and information I provide within the 16 chapters of this book, help you not only survive, but thrive, as a caregiver. Remember, you cannot take care of others, if you, yourself are not healthy. Taking care of yourself and your health is paramount.

While writing this book, I consulted many colleagues, friends, and family members, and the consensus was overwhelming that the need for this information is so greatly necessary. It would have been so helpful for me to have had a book such as this to rely on, when I had first became a caregiver to my grandma. From the bottom of my heart, I hope this book gives you all the tools and resources you will need, to make your experience as painless as possible, so that you can derive some joy and feelings of purpose in your caregiver journey.

Chapter 1
Understanding Dementia

The Brain and Dementia

The brain, easily the most complex object in the known universe, contains almost one hundred billion nerve cells. These nerve cells are responsible for movement, thinking, learning, behavior, hand-eye coordination, breathing, and everything and anything else you can possibly think of.

Until recently, doctors and scientists were only able to study the changes in a person's brain post-mortem. With recent advancements in technology, including MRIs, brain scans, and neurological imaging, we can now understand what happens to the brain in certain diseases that cause it to degenerate and, over time, lose its function.

Understanding this, we can affirm that dementia is caused by neurodegeneration. When the neurons are damaged, they eventually die. Over time (at a rate depending on the person), certain parts of the brain lose their ability to function.

Primarily, the brain is responsible for the following functions:

- Personality
- Memory
- Ordering
- Emotions
- Vision
- Language
- Body Control
- Spatial Awareness
- Behavior

Each of these functions is controlled by one of six specific brain parts:

- Cerebrum
- Cerebellum
- Frontal Lobe
- Parietal Lobe
- Temporal Lobe and Hippocampus
- Occipital Lobe

From recording our actions to regulating our reactions, the brain is a hub that constantly receives stimuli from our six senses. It assimilates the stimuli into information and then coordinates our response to the stimuli through our senses.

The brain forms memories. The ability to store and process these memories is what is called upon throughout our lives, aka our "bank" of knowledge. The brain is also responsible for direct and abstract thoughts, consciousness, personality, and emotions.

Since you are living with someone diagnosed with dementia, you deserve to know how each part of the brain affects this disease - this way, you know who to thank.

Cerebrum

The cerebrum is involved in memory, attention, language, consciousness, thought, senses, and movement. It's the largest part of the brain and is made up of folded grey matter, which gives it a wrinkled look - think of the wrinkly Shar Pei dog.

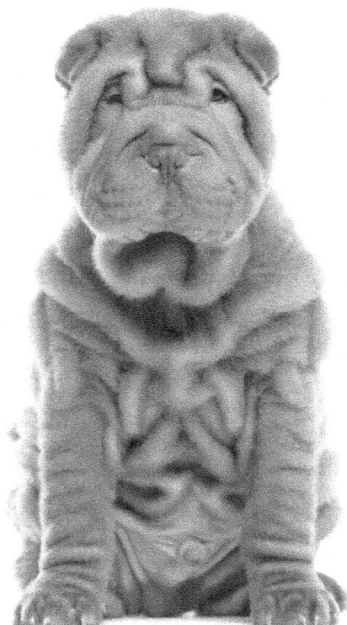

When dementia affects the cerebrum, as it does in the case of Lewy Body Dementia, protein builds up in the grey matter in the form of lumps, harming the nerve cells and causing the patient to hallucinate and zone in and out of consciousness.

Vascular dementia also affects the cerebrum by reducing blood flow, causing brain cells to die, due to a lack of oxygen and nutrition.

Cerebellum

Balance, posture, movements, language, and attention span are all controlled by the cerebellum. Being a progressive disease, dementia causes symptoms to worsen as more brain cells become damaged. By the time the cerebellum is affected, your loved one will have trouble maintaining their balance, using the right words, and paying attention for any length of time.

Frontal Lobe

The frontal lobe is responsible for emotions, personality, and behavior. It's the part of the brain that differentiates between good and bad, as well as predicts the outcome of our actions. It's the part of the brain that inhibits inappropriate social behavior. Whenever you recognize patterns and similarities and differences and contrasts, you can thank your frontal lobe. Also stored in the frontal lobe are our long-term memories.

Some types of dementia that affect the cerebrum, such as frontotemporal dementia, is caused by abnormal lumps of proteins in that part of the brain, damaging nerve cells. As a result of this damage, frontotemporal dementia patients behave inappropriately and uninhibitedly. Don't be surprised by stark personality changes and/or behavior completely uncharacteristic of your loved one.

Parietal Lobe

When you see letters that can form a word, words that can form a sentence, or a math problem that requires solving, your parietal lobe is responsible for their processing. The parietal lobe is also responsible for sensory perception, i.e., knowing where our arms and legs are with respect to the rest of our body. It also allows us to see three-dimensional objects.

Posterior cortical atrophy (a rare form of Alzheimer's), which causes damage to the parietal lobe, affects your loved one's ability to process and perceive objects and their location. Your loved one can lose their sense of connection between body parts, which can result in confusion.

Temporal Lobe

The temporal lobe perceives how you interpret what you see and hear. When it comes to recall, such as recognizing people, things, objects, and places, all of that processing takes place in the temporal lobe. When your loved one experiences issues with language skills, such as word recall and the ability to recognize and remember names of people and various objects, damage to the temporal lobe is a contributing factor.

Hippocampus

The hippocampus, which is a tiny part of the temporal lobe, enables us to form new memories and is credited with our ability to remember such things as names, appointments, directions, places, locations, etc.

There are two proteins that build up in this tiny part of the temporal lobe, causing damage to nerve cells and, albeit slowly, spreading to other parts of the brain. The build-up of these two proteins (amyloid and tau) is responsible for difficulty in remembering things, problems with speech, language, and overall remembrance.

Occipital Lobe

This part of the brain determines how our eyes perceive shapes, colors, and even how objects move around. This lobe processes the stimuli it receives from your eyes.

Damage to the occipital lobe eventually occurs in most types of dementia. Presentation of this damage can appear in your loved one having difficulty understanding and interpreting what they are seeing, and severe damage can alter perception up to the point of causing visual hallucinations.

HUMAN BRAIN ANATOMY

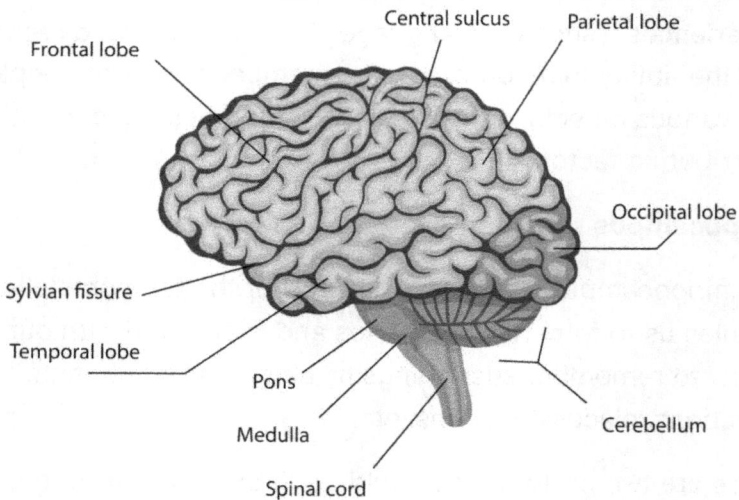

Frontal lobe

Central sulcus

Parietal lobe

Occipital lobe

Sylvian fissure

Temporal lobe

Pons

Medulla

Cerebellum

Spinal cord

If you have come this far (I thank you), you have been introduced to each part of the brain and how it is affected by dementia. Now, it's time for me to share what dementia actually is.

Although understanding the science behind dementia is not necessary to become a caregiver (you don't have to pass an exam), it will be helpful for you to understand what the disease is and its symptoms, stages, and types.

To understand what dementia is, we have to know what dementia is not. Dementia is not a normal part of aging. In fact, one of the widespread yet false beliefs about dementia is that it is the same thing as senility. This leads people to believe that the symptoms of dementia, primarily the decline of mental faculties, are a normal part of aging, which includes the weakening of bones and muscles, stiffening of blood vessels, and age-related memory loss. Another misconception about dementia is that it only affects the elderly. Unfortunately, there are people under the age of 65 being diagnosed with dementia, known as early-onset dementia.

Please do your homework because not all symptoms of mental decline equals dementia. Your loved one could have symptoms parroting those of dementia. These symptoms may come from a condition that is reversible, such as vitamin deficiencies, thyroid issues, hormonal disorders, malnutrition, long-term alcoholism, depression, stroke, brain tumors, or infections. To qualify as dementia, your first step would be to rule out any of these reversible causes and assess if a patient's mental impairment is affecting at least two of the following major brain functions: memory, language, judgment, behavior, or thinking.

Dementia is often mistaken for a single disease, whereas it is actually an umbrella term that encapsulates several medical conditions related to memory loss and the deterioration of related mental abilities, such as cognition and thinking. The term is used for disorders such as Alzheimer's, Vascular Dementia, Lewy Body Dementia, Frontotemporal Dementia, Huntington's Disease, and so on. While dementia is not a particular disease, different diseases can cause dementia.

Dementia is a neurodegenerative disease, which means that it progressively degenerates the nerve cells, resulting in irreparable damage to the brain. Dementia is not curable. For some, its progression can be controlled or slowed down through proper care and medication, but it can not be stopped or reversed. This disease impacts not only you and your loved one's physical and psychological health but can also affect economic and social aspects for both of you.

What Causes Dementia?

The primary cause of dementia is neurodegenerative diseases, which affect the way neurons connect to each other via synapses.

Dementia can also be caused by structural brain disorders, such as subdural hematomas and normal pressure hydrocephalus. Metabolic disorders, such as vitamin B12 deficiency, hypothyroidism, and kidney and liver disorders, can also cause dementia. Toxins, such as lead and mercury, can also cause dementia, as can symptoms related to brain tumors or brain infections. Even medication side effects can be a culprit.

Risk factors contributing to developing dementia:

- Age
- Family history
- Race/ethnicity
- Poor heart health
- Traumatic brain injury
- High blood pressure
- High blood sugar
- Obesity
- Alcohol consumption
- Smoking
- Physical inactivity
- Depression
- Social isolation

Chapter 2
Symptoms of Dementia

Symptoms and Warning Signs

Most of the symptoms are very subtle in the early stages, making it difficult to detect. Furthermore, symptoms differ from person to person, as does each form of dementia.

The most common early symptoms of dementia include:

- Memory loss
- Difficulty performing ordinary tasks
- Disorientation
- Language trouble
- Loss of abstract thinking
- Judgment difficulties
- Change in spatial skills
- Misplacing items

- Change in personality
- Withdrawal from society

If your loved one exhibits one or more of the following **ten warning signs of dementia**, a doctor's consultation is in order.

1. Memory Loss

Some amount of memory loss is natural and expected with age. But, it's when one begins to forget important details and/or appointments, dates, etc., that you should start paying attention and take note of these patterns. If it persists, it very well may be an early symptom of dementia.

2. Difficulty Performing Ordinary Tasks

A person with dementia will not be able to recall all the steps necessary in performing ordinary tasks, whether it relates to driving a car, cooking a meal (including ingredients for their favorite dishes), or washing clothes.

3. Disorientation

Dementia patients can have difficulty orienting themselves, especially when it concerns their location. They can become confused about where they are or where they are going. Sometimes, they believe they are living in the past.

4. Language Trouble

A dementia patient will struggle with more than just finding the right words. They won't be able to recall simple words.

Sometimes, they might even substitute strange words in their place, making it very hard for people to understand what they're saying. The trouble with language is not confined to speaking. Those who suffer from dementia can also have difficulty understanding what others are saying.

5. Loss of Abstract Thinking

Other instances of thinking, include abstract thinking, such as: checking off checklists, doing one's taxes, managing a budget, and keeping one's grocery needs in mind while shopping. Analytical thinking required during specific activities, such as assembling simple items, are also affected by dementia.

6. Judgment Difficulties

A patient with dementia will not be able to handle decisions or make appropriate choices, especially relating to money and finances, which would include paying monthly bills. They might forget that it's cold outside and that they should be wearing warm clothes. They may not recall that they have to put gas in the car when the tank is empty.

7. Change in Spatial Skills

Similarly, spatial skills, such as judging the distance between two cars on the road or perceiving the speed of an oncoming vehicle, are affected adversely by those who suffer from dementia.

8. Misplacing Items

Everyone tends to lose their keys or wallet from time to time. The troubling sign is when a person forgets what the keys are for or why they have a wallet, to begin with.

9. Changes in Personality

Dementia can cause rapid mood swings, confusion, withdrawal from other people, suspicion, paranoia, rudeness, anger, and disinhibition. People who suffer from dementia tend to become more outgoing in instances when their inhibitions are low or, in the alternative, become withdrawn.

10. Withdrawal from Society

Often, dementia causes depression, which can lead to your loved one withdrawing from their favorite activities and lose interest in important relationships. Helping your loved one socialize can be as simple as inviting family and friends over and providing cues and clues to help them join in. Walking, wheeling, or just sitting outside with your loved one offers an opportunity to get outside the house and enjoy the fresh air. Puzzles, card games, and even listening to music can provide the perfect catalyst to stimulate the brain and enjoy some special shared moments together.

A doctor's diagnosis of dementia is not based on the above symptoms alone; it is based on a compilation of the patient's medical history, laboratory tests, a physical check-up, and changes in their day-to-day ability to function. Although your doctor can determine whether or not your loved one has dementia, the difficult aspect of diagnosis, is ascertaining the exact type of dementia, as many symptoms overlap with each other. Specialists, such as neurologists, psychiatrists, and geriatricians, are among the professionals consulted to distinguish between the various types and should be consulted in order to make a proper diagnosis.

Specific Symptoms Related to the Various Forms of Dementia

Alzheimer's disease symptoms include:

- Becoming aloof and anxious
- Repetitive questioning regarding a topic
- Memory-related issues, such as forgetting people's names and faces or the inability to recall something that happened recently
- Becoming confused, which could be exacerbated by new environments
- Inability to come up with the appropriate word while engaged in a conversation. Using inappropriate words or just words that are not relevant to the conversation
- Difficulty dealing with money, especially in social settings. An example of this can be displayed when your loved one is at a shop and attempting to pay for their purchase at the register
- Inability to plan and organize

Although Alzheimer's is the most prevalent type of dementia, vascular dementia is not far behind on the list of the most common forms of dementia. Many people are afflicted with both Alzheimer's and vascular dementia. This combination is termed mixed dementia.

If your loved one has only vascular dementia, memory loss may not be one of the early symptoms. The symptoms of vascular dementia can seem to appear from nowhere, and these symptoms can worsen overnight. In the alternative, symptoms may take months and years to develop.

Vascular Dementia symptoms include:

- Stroke-like symptoms, which can include muscular weakness and/or one-sided body paralysis. In either case, urgent medical care would be recommended and highly advisable
- Difficulty in moving, which could be seen in such activities as walking, sitting (sitting down and rising up), getting in and out of bed, etc.
- Difficulty thinking, which would be recognized by a reduced attention span, trouble with reasoning, and an inability to plan, etc.
- Mood swings and shifts that tend to gravitate toward depression

Lewy Body Dementia symptoms include:

- Periods of alertness followed by periods of drowsiness
- Fluctuating levels of disconcertment
- Hallucinations (visual)
- Slowed physical movements
- Repeatedly fainting or falling
- Sleep Disturbances

Frontotemporal Dementia symptoms include:

- Changes in personality
- Reduced sensitivity to others' feelings. This can appear as disinterest or coldness
- Inability to exhibit social awareness. This can be displayed by dirty jokes, tactlessness, apathy, social withdrawal, social awkwardness, etc.

- Obsessive behavior, observed by binge eating, binge drinking, washing hands, checking door locks, etc.
- Difficulty with language

Chapter 3
Stages of Dementia

While most people think of dementia in terms of three phases —early, middle, and late, also known as mild, moderate, and severe—we are going to take a deeper dive into the world of dementia and examine its seven stages. My objective is to provide you with the tools you will find necessary to better understand the journey we are about to begin. Knowledge is power! You wouldn't send a soldier into a battle without proper ammunition and protection. Likewise, you need to be armed with knowledge so that you can understand both the stages and symptoms of this disease.

Each form of dementia advances at its own rate. However, the symptoms can be generalized into phases and stages.

Pre-dementia: A pre-dementia patient is still able to function independently. Their memory loss and loss of cognitive function are not yet obvious. The symptoms of pre-dementia often mimic senior moments.

Moderate Dementia: Your loved one's personality is beginning to show symptoms of this disease. These symptoms become apparent in their everyday behavior. At this time, you will need to address your loved one's need for part or full-time caregiving - so get ready.

Severe Dementia: This final phase is where severe cognitive impairment takes place, as well as the loss of physical abilities.

The Global Deterioration Scale is used by healthcare providers. This scale distinguishes dementia progression and divides it into seven stages. This allows you, the caregiver, and other healthcare providers a way to track your loved one's overall health and symptoms. The seven stages include:

Stage 1: No Cognitive Impairment

In this beginning stage, the symptoms are so mild or non-existent that your loved one is able to go about their day without any signs of decline in cognitive functions. Actually, when in one of the first three stages of dementia, symptoms may not be apparent and therefore, not diagnosed.

Stage 2: Very Mild Cognitive Impairment

Your loved one will begin to have memory lapses. Some of these may include forgetting where they put their keys, remembering a person's name, forgetting what they got up to get, etc. This is a difficult stage to diagnose because many seniors can display these forms of impairment, and is considered to be plain, old age-related forgetfulness.

Stage 3: Mild Cognitive Impairment

At this stage, cognitive impairment becomes more noticeable to you, the caregiver, as well as other family members and friends. Your loved one may forget to go to scheduled appointments. They will have forgotten to mark their calendar or forget to look at it. They can lose things around the house and spend hours looking for these items and become very frustrated doing so.

Your loved one can get turned around while out and about. If they are still driving, it's probably time to take their keys. If they make a wrong turn or forget where they are, or where they are going, they can easily become lost and confused, even scared. This is known as the perfect storm, a recipe for disaster- a car accident.

If your loved one is still working, they will, at this stage, begin to experience performance-related issues. Losing the ability to recall appropriate words becomes a constant problem, as does repeating the same conversation over and over and over again.

Stage 4: Moderate Cognitive Impairment

Marked cognitive impairment and personality shifts are prevalent at this stage of dementia. Symptoms that mark this stage include social withdrawal, reduced responsiveness, mood swings, reduced intelligence, difficulty performing routine tasks, and increased forgetfulness. Your loved one may be in denial and refute the possibility that they may have dementia and try to cover it up whenever possible.

Stage 5: Moderately Severe Cognitive Impairment

This mid-stage of dementia is characterized by an increased difficulty in carrying out normal daily tasks, to the point that a person is incapable of performing them at all, by the end of this stage. This stage can go on for up to four years. As the symptoms become more pronounced, your loved one will require more upfront caregiving and supervision. You must understand that no two people are exactly the same. At any time going forward, your loved one may require constant supervision.

Stage 6: Severe Cognitive Impairment

At this stage, your loved one will need full-time assistance to deal with daily activities. These include getting up, going to the bathroom, dressing, eating, and everything else you do during the day, including preparing for sleep. Your loved one might have difficulty falling and staying asleep, which can be exacerbated by incontinence and urinary tract infections (UTIs). Your loved one can exhibit signs of aggression and anxiety. Huge personality changes, including delusions and paranoia, will increase with more pronounced memory loss. There can come a time when your loved one is unable to recognize their loved ones, including you, the caregiver. Understand this can happen, and sadly oftentimes does - be prepared.

You, acting as caregiver, should begin monitoring your loved one's activities of daily life (ADL) and instrumental activities of daily life (IADL), in order to track these changes, which will appear in this sixth stage. The activities of daily life (ADL) include eating, drinking, bathing, reading, personal grooming, and cooking. The instrumental activities of daily life (IADL) include specifics, like using the phone to answer calls and call others, shopping for groceries, managing medication, managing finances (including bills), and housekeeping.

Stage 7: Very Severe Cognitive Impairment

This stage is considered end-stage dementia and is marked by your loved one's complete inability to function. All verbal and movement abilities are lost—voluntary movements like chewing, swallowing, and drinking become severely difficult, if not impossible. Eventually, involuntary body functions, such as breathing, cease.

Chapter 4
Diagnosis

Diagnosis and Prognosis

Healthcare professionals diagnose dementia by first asking relevant questions pertaining to the patient's medical history. This is followed by a physical exam, a mental status exam, lab tests, and imaging tests.

When all this information is put together, your doctor can determine if your loved one's loss of mental capabilities is caused by dementia or not. Even though dementia is not a treatable disease, it's vital that you know what type of dementia your loved one has, so that proper medications can be prescribed and other treatments suggested, which can improve your loved one's behavior and mood; this will also be very helpful to you, as the caregiver.

Patient History

The diagnosis begins with your doctor asking questions about your loved one's medical history. Your doctor should ask pertinent questions, such as when the symptoms began and what your loved one's overall medical journey has been like. As I already mentioned, some patients are in denial and won't admit or believe they have dementia. You will find that some of your family members can buy into this denial. This can occur because there is so much unawareness and stigma associated with the disease.

Physical Exam

A physical examination rules out other diseases that might be treatable. It can identify if the symptoms are actually arising from other diseases and illnesses that can mimic dementia-related symptoms, such as stroke, kidney, or heart failure. Check-ups can also reveal if a medication or combination of medications are causing the symptoms.

Neurological Examination

A neurological exam should include looking at the patient's sensory function, balance, reflexes, motor functions, and movement. This will enable the doctor to determine whether their symptoms align with those of dementia.

Cognitive and Neuropsychological Testing

These tests measure the patient's language skills, math skills, memory, spatial skills, and mental function. A patient with dementia will show changes in their executive functions, such as analytical thinking, memory, and performing automated tasks.

This is a very specialized and time-consuming process and is handled by a trained neuropsychologist.

Tests like the Mini-Mental State Examination (MMSE) allow doctors to assess the cognitive skills of their patients. Tests like the MMSE of the Montreal Cognitive Assessment (MoCA) examine a patient's memory, attention, orientation, and ability to name things, understand verbal cues, or draw a complex shape.

Other tests that doctors can conduct can help specify the exact type and cause of cognitive impairment. These tests include:

Brain Scans

While doctors do use brain scans to identify tumors, strokes, and other neurological disorders, they also use these scans to identify dementia. The brain's outer layer starts to degenerate in several forms of dementia, which is usually visible in a brain scan.

The most common types of scans used are magnetic resonance imaging (MRI) and computed tomographic (CT) scans. CT scans utilize X-rays to decipher the brain's structure. These scans show the presence of atrophy, strokes, ischemia, blood vessel damage, hydrocephalus, and subdural hematomas. MRIs, on the other hand, utilize magnetic fields and radio waves to detect the hydrogen atoms present within the tissues of the brain.

Laboratory Tests

Doctors use an array of lab tests to assist in making a diagnosis of dementia. These tests usually serve to rule out other conditions that might be causing dementia-like symptoms, such as a vitamin deficiency or hormonal imbalance.

These tests include: a blood glucose test, complete blood count, drug/alcohol test, cerebrospinal fluid analysis, thyroid and thyroid-stimulating hormone level analysis, B12 level, and kidney and liver tests.

Psych Eval

A psychiatric evaluation may be deemed necessary if depression or other mental health conditions are contributing to symptoms that look like dementia.

Pre-symptomatic Testing

Even though there aren't many tests that can ascertain if a patient will get dementia in the future, in some cases, genetic defects can be detected early on, such as in the case of Huntington's.

Assembling Your Healthcare Team

You, your loved one, and other family members will most likely have a million questions. Some of the most asked questions relate to medications, care, what to avoid, and the type of specialists you should consult.

Your healthcare team will evolve over time, depending on the needs of your loved one. Your basic team should include the following doctors, who should be able to assist and support you through the various stages of this disease.

Primary Care Physician

Your first step should be to consult with your primary care physician, if you suspect your loved one is beginning to have issues with their memory. Your primary care physician, if he or she has diagnosed your loved one with dementia, should be your point person, and he or she should be willing to accept the responsibility for coordinating your loved one's treatment.

Neurologist and Neuropsychologist

A neurologist is a doctor who specializes in the diagnosis, treatment, and management of disorders of the brain and nervous system, including Parkinson's, dementia, epilepsy, stroke, and cluster headaches.

The neuropsychologist is a psychologist who specializes in the brain's cognitive functions, such as memory, language, and attention. They conduct tests that assess memory, concentration, language skills, and problem-solving capacity.

Geriatrician

A geriatrician is a physician who specializes in treating the elder population. Your geriatrician will be invaluable, as they will be able to collaborate with the primary care physician and, together, can help in managing your loved one's care.

Geriatric Psychiatrist

Geriatric psychiatrists specialize in the behavioral and emotional condition of elders and are often consulted with regard to the management of associated behavioral issues. Geriatric psychiatrists, unlike the geropsychologist, can prescribe medications as needed to treat these mental health issues. Such issues include anger, sleep deprivation, depression, paranoia, agitation, etc.

Geropsychologist

A geropsychologist provides therapy and counseling for elders. This physician focuses on sociological, emotional, psychological, neurological, and physical issues pertaining to the elderly.

Occupational Therapist

An occupational therapist identifies difficulties with regard to independent functions and everyday activities. Various forms of occupational therapy interventions, such as memory aids, can be a huge help in adapting both you and your loved one to their ever-changing world.

Audiologist

The audiologist can become a significant member of your loved one's healthcare team.

An audiologist is capable of identifying, assessing, and managing hearing disorders. If not consulted, these issues, coupled with the issue of balance, can further lead to social withdrawal and depression.

Ophthalmologist

An ophthalmologist treats all conditions related to the eyes. Because the retina and optic nerve are part of the brain tissue that extends outside the braincase, eyes can be affected by dementia. Accordingly, an ophthalmologist should be considered when assembling your healthcare team.

Nurses

Specialized dementia nurses, also known as admiral nurses in the United Kingdom, help family members manage the complex needs of your loved one, facilitate your loved one to remain active and independent for longer, can assess important issues in patient safety, and also can be instrumental in managing behavioral issues that your loved one will continue to face.

Doctor's Visits - What Questions to Ask and How to Stay Organized

Here's a checklist that I hope you will find helpful when structuring your healthcare team and preparing for your doctor visits.

If you are computer savvy, you can CLICK here, input this site: https://bit.ly/3MenDD9, or scan the QR code below and download the medical binder that I have created for you.

Don't worry; I haven't forgotten those of you who may not have access or feel comfortable using a computer. I am arming you with a step-by-step blueprint, so that you can get organized.

A 3-ring binder with dividers or a planner with tabs, works well to house all of your information. This will prove helpful to you in maintaining all of your information and keeping your records together in one place.

The main partitions in your binder should include the following:

Emergency Contacts

Includes telephone numbers of:

- Primary caregiver
- Secondary/tertiary caregivers
- Immediate household or family members
- Doctors
- Therapists
- Nurses
- Care facilities
- Other peripheral contacts that may be called upon, such as close friends, empathetic family members, who've been helpful in the past, and neighbors

Medical History

The medical history portion of the binder should include:

- Current diagnosis
- Other medical conditions
- Past surgeries
- Presence of metal in their body, i.e.: plates, rods, artificial joints, etc.
- Pacemakers
- If there's a Do Not Resuscitate (DNR) Order, include that document in the legal section of your binder and write DNR on the top right corner of the cover page

Medications

This list would include:

- Name
- Dosage (how much and what time of day to take)

- Start date and end date (if the medication is discontinued)
- Reactions or adverse effects (this should be explicit)
- With or without Food

Allergies

You should include any reactions to food or medications.

Doctor visits

In this section of the binder, you should include:

- Monthly calendar to keep track of doctor visits
- List of questions that you have asked or will ask doctors on visits and a compiled list of notes that you've made after those questions were answered
- Include any new plans and visits to the doctor, as well as, any changes to treatment plans and medications
- Medications can be a case of trial and error. During your visit, be sure to inquire about any changes or adjustments regarding doses
- Discuss behavioral changes your loved one has experienced and inquire if any treatments or medications are available
- Ask about potential side effects and if necessary, what to look out for in terms of side-effect symptoms
- Inquire as to whether or not there is a particular time that the medications should be taken. You need to know if the medication should be given with or without food
- Have the doctor advise you on expectations regarding the period of time necessary for the medication to take effect

- Is there a duration of time wherein the medication is no longer effective or safe

Legal Documents

I will cover this topic in detail in chapter 12; however, there are some necessary legal documents that you should include in your binder, including, but not limited to:

- Power of attorney
- Power of attorney for healthcare
- Advance directives such as a living will or trust
- Do not resuscitate order (DNR)
- Insurance information

Chapter 5

Treatment and Care

One of my patients, Rachel, spoke of her experience as a caregiver for her father, who was diagnosed with early-onset Alzheimer's, when Rachel had just turned 24. The emotional dissonance that Rachel experienced after learning about her father's diagnosis rattled her. Her immediate reaction was one of denial. Rachel could not believe her father had dementia. Her denial soon transformed, and all she could think of was how she was going to be able to care for her father. Rachel's mother had passed away a few years earlier, and her father was always there to care for her, her mom, and her siblings. There was no doubt she was going to do whatever was necessary to care for her father, in his time of need. It was clear to Rachel that their roles were being reversed and Rachel knew it was up to her to take the reins.

Rachel asked the doctor many questions, and it became clear to her that in order to take on this role, she needed to understand everything possible about this disease. Having graduated from college, Rachel was in the prime of her life:

dating, working, traveling; she had it all and was as happy as could be. She had never imagined a world where her life could take such a 180-degree turn. Although Rachel was the youngest of her three siblings, due to personal issues, living arrangements, and responsibilities, it became apparent that Rachel was the only one who could possibly take on the responsibility and role of caregiver for her father.

Although Rachel's life would be turned upside down, and she never imagined having to be a primary caregiver, she was going to do what she had to, in order to take care of her father. As she began to share her feelings with me, Rachel expressed that she always dreamt of her father walking her down the aisle at her wedding. She also had always envisioned having a family and pictured her father as a grandpa, with her children in his arms and them playing together, as he always did with her and her siblings. He was the best father, and she knew he would make the very best grandfather. She said that she was devastated, by the realization that her dreams and visions were no longer going to be a reality.

It took a while, but once she came to terms with the situation, she did not allow it to deter her. She made the decision to appreciate each moment she had with her dad, cherishing the time she spent with him and the stories and conversations they shared. Her memories of her wonderful childhood and the many great times they shared, helped turn her sadness into gratitude. Rachel's story and the intent of her message became one of thankfulness and optimism. Yours can be as well. Rachel equipped herself with a wealth of information and gained the knowledge necessary to care for her father so that she was able to understand what he was going through and the treatments and care he would need along the way. By doing so, Rachel was better able to anticipate future behavioral and medical challenges and was able to establish a framework to collaborate with her healthcare team. Arming herself with this knowledge and facing the reality of what the future would be without sugarcoating it, ultimately gave her the strength to deal with the challenges as they arose head-on. My hope, is that by hearing these stories and reading this book, you, too, will feel empowered and be able to embrace the care you provide for your loved one, with gratitude and optimism.

Although dementia is not curable, to date, there are treatments available that can help in controlling and managing the symptoms and, if you are lucky, can even slow down the progression of the disease.

Treatments are usually based on the symptoms your loved one presents. As mentioned, assembling a team of doctors who coordinate with each other is a must. Varying treatments available for dementia include managing symptoms and slowing progression.

Medications Available to Manage Symptoms

Cognitive decline is inevitable as dementia progresses because the connections among brain cells are lost as the brain cells die. There are drugs available, which I list below, that can stabilize symptoms, thereby lessening their intensity by affecting the chemicals involved in carrying messages between brain cells. Please remember that these drugs can neither reverse nor stop the damage that has already taken place.

Cholinesterase Inhibitors are a group of medications that prevent the breakdown of the chemical messenger known as acetylcholine, which is responsible for memory, learning, and judgment. Donepezil (Aricept), Rivastigmine (Exelon), and Galantamine (Razadyne) are amongst the most commonly prescribed medications in this class.

Another chemical messenger, known as Glutamate, enables the brain to process information. Glutamate regulators such as **Memantine (Namenda)** help to improve attention span, reasoning, language, and memory.

There are medications available that combine cholinesterase inhibitors and glutamate regulators: Donepezil + Memantine (Namzaric), which has been approved for mild to severe dementia symptoms.

Hallucinations, sleep disturbance, agitation, and delusions are examples of non-cognitive symptoms known to be associated with dementia. There are many drugs available that can help control and manage these symptoms. They are:

Suvorexant (Belsomra) is a medication that has been approved by the FDA to treat insomnia. This drug inhibits the activity of orexin, a neurotransmitter involved in the sleep-wake cycle. Information regarding this drug's benefits relating to insomnia in mild to moderate Alzheimer's disease patients has been found through research by the manufacturer and is provided in the patient package insert.

Atypical Antipsychotics, typically used to treat bipolar disorder and schizophrenia, have been found to have benefits in treating dementia-related behavior by targeting the serotonin and dopamine chemical pathways in the brain. Research and studies have demonstrated that this class of medications can be used to alleviate agitation, hallucinations, and delusions. Two of the most commonly used medications in this class include Haloperidol (Haldol) and Brexpiprazole (Rexulti).

As with all medications, there are potential side effects. It is important to discuss the pros and cons (side effects and benefits) of each medication with your healthcare team. Once a medication is determined to be beneficial, it is of the utmost importance to both understand and follow your doctor's and pharmacist's instructions, to minimize any negative side effects and interactions. Examples would include whether to take the medication after eating, or on an empty stomach, the time of day (morning or night), and the prescribed dosage. If the existing dosage is causing negative side effects, the doctor may be able to lower the dose and, or switch the medication. Finding the right medication and the proper dosage to treat the symptom may only be discovered by trial and error, but eventually, you should be able to find the right fit.

Medications Available that Help to Slow Progression:

There are already medications on the market that have been known to slow the progression of the disease. Research and testing have shown that these drugs can slow down the progression of dementia by tackling the underlying biology responsible for the disease's progression. These medications can potentially slow down the decline of thinking, memory, and function.

Beta-amyloid is a protein that deteriorates the brain's function by accumulating into plaques. **Amyloid-targeting treatments** attach to and remove these beta-amyloids. This type of treatment is helpful to people in the early stages of dementia. This may provide your loved one with more time to remain physically active, as well as curtail memory loss and disorientation. **Aducanumab** and **Lecanemab** are forms of intravenous (IV) therapies that serve to remove beta-amyloids from the brain. Both are FDA-approved treatments for dementia.

Alternative Remedies and Therapies

Many alternative holistic remedies are available, which we will delve into in greater detail in chapter 14.

Cognitive Stimulation Therapy (CST)

Cognitive stimulation therapy (CST) is an evidence-based treatment for people with mild to moderate dementia, which involves group activities, exercises, and tasks that can help to improve cognitive function, language ability, analytical skills, and memory skills.

Cognitive Rehabilitation

A trained professional (therapist) will assist the patient by using memory exercises, problem-solving games, and other mental exercises that have proved to be beneficial by utilizing those parts of the brain affected by dementia. It provides a better indication of what stage your loved one is in, and the progression of the disease.

Reminiscence Therapy

One of the more fun therapies, is known as reminiscence therapy, wherein you are spending time with your loved one, talking and sharing special moments and times in their life. Oftentimes, your loved one will be able to recall memorable events, their favorite people, their favorite songs, movies, and books. This can include taking out a scrapbook and having them identify different people and places, which can jog their long-term memory. This form of therapy can be a great tool in diverting depression and improving moods, even if it's short-term.

Occupational Therapy

An occupational therapist is the person to go to who can help to ensure that your home is safe for your loved one and may recommend environmental modifications, when necessary. They will make suggestions and even assist you in rearranging your home to minimize accidents, as well as teach both you and your loved one new ways to handle daily chores/activities —hint: the less clutter, the better.

In this chapter, we discussed various types of treatments available for dementia, including different therapies, medications, and environmental modifications. Now, let's review the various behavioral issues and how to manage them best.

Chapter 6
Managing and Understanding Common Behavioral Issues

Geriatric psychiatrists and nurses can help manage behavioral issues that commonly arise with the help of medication and strategies.

Before we look at some of the major behavioral issues and learn how to manage them, I would like to share another one of my patient's recent experiences, that she went through when her father was diagnosed with dementia. Her name is Mary.

Mary thought that she was ready. She felt that she was prepared for the physical and mental toll, dementia would have on herself, her father, and their family. She soon realized how unprepared she actually was. Without any notice, her father's behavior changed drastically. Overnight, he became very aggressive, and there were sexual undertones. She told me that one moment he was sweet and loving, and the next moment was confusing her with her mother - his wife. She said that he would use inappropriate language and gestures, both of which made her feel so uncomfortable. Mary became extremely overwhelmed and was finding it more and more difficult to cope with these behavioral changes.

There's no doubt about it, dementia and its various forms are extremely tough for your loved one, as well as for you, the caregiver. Your loved one can become angry, agitated, anxious, depressed, and even act out sexually. Actions can run the gamut; from wandering, repeating things, hallucinating, hoarding things, etc.

It's important to remember that all of these behaviors and actions are beyond your loved one's control. As the primary caregiver, you will be facing these challenges, and unfortunately, they will expand and progress, as does the disease. Being prepared and having an understanding of these behavioral issues will help you to navigate your own feelings of frustration, anger, bitterness, and depression. Since we are only human, feeling these emotions can not be avoided. However, how you deal with them can be controlled and make all the difference. I will share some coping and management strategies to help you tackle these issues throughout the varying stages.

Nonpharmacological Strategies for Managing Behavioral Issues:

Communication

Many behavioral issues arise out of sheer confusion. When disconcerted, your loved one may act out and become agitated. Effective communication is key to helping prevent confusion, and you can do so by:

- Allow them sufficient time to respond to a question
- Talk to them in a reassuring voice
- Avoid negative words and tone
- Help them to identify you and others if and when name recognition becomes a challenge
- Assist your loved one in finding ways to express themselves when words become a challenge

Simplifying the Environment

Another contributing factor that can lead to confusion can result from an overwhelming environment. Removing clutter can help simplify this problem. This includes removing all unnecessary objects. Placing visual reminders and cues around the house, such as arrows pointing to the bathroom, their name and/or picture on their bedroom door, and colorful tape indicating a step, are all tools that can aid in making your loved one's daily life safer and easier.

Caregiver Education and Support

As said before, information is power. As the caregiver, it is important for you to understand and educate yourself - so, keep reading, you are right on track! Having professional assistance and the love and support of friends and family is huge. Remember, taking care of yourself while caring for your loved one is especially essential and is so important that I cover this subject extensively, in chapter 15.

Simplifying Tasks

There will come a time when your loved one will become unable to perform ordinary tasks on their own. Consider simplifying these once simple tasks, by reconstructing them into smaller, more simplified steps. Each step can have a verbal and/or tactile prompt, which will assist your loved one and allow them to achieve success.

Activities

It is important to allow your loved one to tap into their remaining abilities, which would provide them with the opportunity to engage in previous interests. By providing a structured routine, they can continue to assist with some tasks that will allow your loved one to feel helpful. Examples of such activities, can include: washing the dishes, folding the laundry, and helping in the kitchen, i.e., mixing batter, setting the table, etc. These simple activities provide your loved one the opportunity to feel included, which can redirect their energy and mental faculties in a positive direction. Sometimes, being left alone sitting in a chair with nothing to do and no one to talk to can make your loved one feel anxious, confused, or angry.

Develop an Evening and Bedtime Routine

It is important to establish a nighttime routine to assist with a good night's sleep and help to avoid a major behavioral issue, known as sundowning. Sundowning, presents with your loved one exhibiting heightened restlessness, anxiety, disorientation, and confusion. It has been given its name because it usually occurs after the sun goes down. As dementia can often upset a person's sleep cycle, do your best to eliminate stimulating activities and foods that contain caffeine and sugar in the evening. In general, too much stimulation should be avoided. On the other hand, it is important that you provide some sort of physical activity for your loved one throughout the day. We do not want them to become listless or board, nor do we want their body to atrophy; but as the day goes on, and night approaches, they should begin to relax in preparation for bedtime. Consider reading a book or watching a relaxing television program together - not the news, especially these days.

Eating Healthy

Limiting your loved one's intake of sugar, caffeine, processed foods, etc., throughout the day is not only important for their health but will also minimize restlessness and anxiety. Eating a healthy diet will help your loved one to be more relaxed, calmer, and ready for a good night's sleep. Chocolate, cakes, cookies, and various forms of candy are commonly everyone's favorite treats. However, they prove to be one of the biggest culprits in robbing your loved one of good mental and physical health and contribute to behavioral issues. Be sure to be cognisant that the food and snacks you offer are healthy alternatives, and do your best to serve foods that are sugar-free when possible. If you can't avoid sugar altogether, use as little as possible, do not use artificial sweeteners; instead do your best to opt for recipes where you can substitute sugar with dates, monk fruit, coconut sugar, stevia, etc. Hopefully, these alternatives will satisfy your loved one's cravings.

Anger and Aggression

As each stage progresses, you will encounter changes in your loved one's personality. 30% of dementia patients lash out at their caregivers and family members. Please, don't take this personally. It has nothing to do with you; you are not the cause of their anger. Aggression is one of the most common symptoms of dementia. More often than not, there is no rhyme or reason; however, there can be underlying causes. The best way to deal with anger and aggressive behavior, is to understand the cause, so that you are able to address it properly.

Some of the most common causes include:

- Disturbed sleep
- Constipation
- Diarrhea
- Pain
- Depression
- Stress
- Anxiety

Examples of underlying causes are:

- Sudden change in routine
- Displacement from a familiar place
- Being surrounded by new people
- Loss-coping, the inability to be independent, unable to go places or do the things they once could
- Loud noise (can cause confusion)
- Overwhelming situations (large groups)
- Control issues - being told when and how to do things: taking a bath, dressing, eating, taking medication, etc.
- Social isolation
- Side-effects of medication
- Physical discomfort - soiled diaper/underwear
- Overstimulation

How would you like me to give you a few tips and tricks to help you deal with and manage anger and aggressive behavior? *I assume your answer to be YES*, and so, here we go:

Sit back and try to relax, but you know that there is a caveat to that. You must make sure that this allowance puts neither you, nor your loved one, in any physical danger.

Frustration can oftentimes lead to feelings of anger and aggression. Your loved one may not be able to verbally express their feelings. Conversely, you may not accurately understand what it is they are trying to communicate. It's important that you do not become frustrated. You must try and understand what they are going through, and instead of reacting negatively, show empathy, even though it might be difficult to do. At all times, keep your cool, count to 10, BREATH, and remind yourself that patience is a virtue. Believe me, I know this is no easy task. However, succeeding will move you one step further to sainthood. 😇

Rule out any physical reasons for their aggression by doing a quick examination to assess whether or not they have any bumps or bruises, which can be a factor in their aggressive behavior. Try to use a calming, reassuring, and gentle voice when speaking to your loved one or asking questions to ascertain if anything is hurting them and or making them uncomfortable. Depending upon your loved one's stage of dementia, they may be communicative or non-communicative, and therefore, you might need to touch areas of their body and ask, does this hurt? Or observe pain through their reaction to your touch.

Distraction is a fabulous tool to employ because by helping your loved one focus on something other than their source of anger or aggression, you can de-escalate their behavior. I would suggest finding a topic of discussion they are interested in, or an activity that they enjoy doing. Finding happy, joyful ways to distract them could be as simple as putting on some music they love, or turning the TV to their favorite program.

I would suggest avoiding physical forms of comfort (hugging) while they are in the throes of their anger. Doing so could serve to heighten their anger and become a danger to either you or your loved one.

If all of these tips and tricks prove unsuccessful and your loved one is unable to calm down, it is important that you stop and assess your situation. You must ensure the safety of you and your loved one at all times. If you can not achieve this on your own, know that you can reach out for help. You do not have to go this alone. Don't be afraid to ask friends or other family members for help. If you are lucky, you have that one person who lives nearby, who has a magical relationship with your loved one, and just the sight of them can mitigate the calamity. If you have no one to turn to, remember you still have avenues for assistance. If finances permit, there are a multitude of agencies that provide all levels of care from trained professionals. If the situation escalates and becomes an emergency, call 911 (or your country's emergency number). Be sure to inform the responder that your loved one has dementia and is exhibiting extremely aggressive behavior and that you are concerned for your and their safety.

As hard as it is, do not admonish your loved one during their outburst. This is one of the hardest mistakes not to make as a caregiver, and it happens all the time. It is very difficult to be non-reactive because, after all, we are only human. Compare it to having a baby or a child who is in the midst of a tantrum and multiply it by 100. Just as a baby or young child might not be capable of understanding why they are acting the way they are, such is true for your loved one with dementia. They are not able to understand and may not even realize their actions. I want you to understand that living with the person you love who has turned into someone you no longer know (a total stranger) is both emotionally and physically taxing. You're doing great; this is a very hard job, and you deserve to be rewarded. Give yourself a great big hug and be proud of what you are doing; you're earning your wings.

Sexual and Intimate Behavioral Changes

As dementia causes degeneration of brain cells, it also affects sexual desires, sexual behavior, and inhibitions, resulting in behavioral changes. Three main aspects are:

1. **Reduced Sex Drive**

If your loved one is your partner, or if you're privy to information about their sexual drive in a caregiving capacity, you may notice that their sexual desire has suddenly plummeted. It could be a symptom of the disease or, more commonly, an indication that they're experiencing side effects from medication or experiencing depression. With the treatment of depression and medication adjustment, their sexual desire may come back.

2. **Increased Sex Drive**

Conversely, your loved one may experience an increased sex drive, as many patients experience a heightened sexual desire resulting from this disease.

3. **Inappropriate Behavior**

Dementia affects the part of the brain that is responsible for inhibition. It can cause your loved one to stop conforming to societal norms and engage in inappropriate behavior.

Try to understand the underlying reason for their behavior. Sometimes, no matter how much you try, there is no rhyme or reason, as there could be multiple reasons for sudden and unexplained sexual advances. One of which could be a desire for affection, which doesn't necessarily indicate a desire for sex. This can be mediated with the help of gentle physical touch and cuddling.

The following tips may be helpful in managing sexual behavior:

- Try to avoid environments that exacerbate sexual behavior, such as overstimulating places or crowded rooms
- Do your best to distract them by redirecting their attention, give them a snack, or put their favorite tv show on - use your imagination
- Eliminate or at the least limit alcohol intake, as alcohol decreases inhibitions
- In the case of mistaken identity, such as demonstrated in the story I shared with you about Mary and her father, you can attempt to remind your loved one who you are (or the person they are mistakenly identifying)
- Your loved one may begin to touch themselves inappropriately in public. If possible, try and communicate to them that what they are doing is not okay, and if that is not successful, you can take them

out of the situation and move them into a more private area. If you are home, take them to their room

Wandering

If your loved one is mobile, wandering can happen at any time for any reason, or for no reason at all. However, excessive stimulation, stress, and anger can exacerbate this serious problem. What makes this so scary, is that your loved one can wander off without anyone noticing. One minute, they are here, and the next minute, they're gone.

Amy, one of my friends, has a grandfather who has severe dementia. One day, he got up at the crack of dawn and left the house while everybody was sleeping. She told me that when she got up, she went into the kitchen and, not seeing her grandfather at the kitchen table, said, "Where is Grandpa?" Her mother looked at her brother, and then they looked at her father, and they realized that Grandpa was missing. Assuming that her grandfather was still asleep, her mom went into his bedroom to wake him up and came back into the kitchen with her hands in the air, saying Grandpa was gone. He wasn't in the bathroom, he wasn't in his bed, and they realized he wasn't in the house. They immediately went outside, each going in a different direction, looking for Grandpa. They checked with neighbors. No one had seen him.

Her grandfather had not driven for years, so they knew he couldn't have gone far. However, after hours of searching to no avail, they decided it was time to call the police. They also contacted other family members and friends who joined them in their search. At the end of the day, no one had found him, and they were petrified, not knowing if he was dead or alive.

This went on the entire day, and fortunately, after dark, a kind stranger knocked on the door, bringing her grandfather home. He told Amy and her family that he found her grandfather sitting on a bench at a nearby bus stop, several blocks from their house, waiting for a bus to take him home. They had no way of knowing what he did during those 12 hours and were thankful that he had no money with him to get on the bus; it was a miracle. They couldn't understand how he could have gone the whole day without eating, drinking, or going to the bathroom - we will never know. Somehow, although he was alone, there must have been some divine intervention because he seemed none the worse for ware. This was a total mystery - one that will never be solved.

Amy told me that they consulted with their doctor, who made several referrals to specialists who deal with these dementia-related issues. In the end, they reviewed all the information they gathered, as well as the suggestions provided, which led them to make the following changes in their home and lifestyle:

- They reduced the amount and level of noise in the home
- They agreed to avoid having any confrontations when Grandpa was in the room
- They replaced their simple locks and alarmed their windows and doors so they would know if any doors or windows were opened

Amy and her family were lucky, and their story had a happy ending. This is not always the case. Wandering is a very serious issue, and you, the caregiver, should be proactive instead of reactive - you'll get a lot fewer grey hairs.

There are many gadgets and apps available to alert you of movement and help you get wandering under better control. I am providing a list of links to sources that will provide you with such tools. If you are reading the ebook, you can access it by clicking HERE, or if you are reading the print version, scan the QR code below with your phone.

Repetitive Actions

If it's not already happening, your loved one will repeat the same thing over and over and over, or ask you the same question a million times. Again, it is hard not to lose your patience and become frustrated, but for both of your sakes, understand that this is not a deliberate action. It is possible that your loved one may no longer be able to remember things in the short term, and drawing attention to this issue, will just make matters worse. If you become upset and or frustrated, your loved one will most probably also get upset and frustrated, which won't do either of you any favors. Although your loved one has no way to control their behavior, you do.

Patience and empathy will give you a big bang for your buck. Telling them over and over again that they already asked you something, or telling them that you already told them (don't you remember?), will potentially confuse them and most probably will make them feel bad and embarrassed, which will not gain you anything positive, rather will create more confusion, frustration, and angst.

Hallucinations

One of my patients, Cindy, told me about her grandmother, who was in the late stage of dementia and was hallucinating on a regular basis. She told me that her grandma would think that her mother (her grandmother's mother) was still alive and saw her around the house all the time. Cindy told me that her grandma would talk to her mother as if she was actually there, whether she was watching TV, or at the dinner table, and it was beginning to really spook her. I advised Cindy to speak with her grandmother's doctor, as hallucinations are a common dementia-related symptom.

If your loved one is hallucinating, I strongly urge you to consult with their doctor - sooner rather than later. Their doctor can prescribe medications, specifically designed to address this symptom. You can create a calm and stimulus-free environment (think spa lounge) where they can relax and chill; remove objects or furniture they can trip on or over while walking; reassure them that you are there for them and that they're safe (remember, all hallucinations are not benign, some can be extremely scary); divert their attention elsewhere: play their favorite song, show them pictures, read them a book, watch TV, etc.

Hoarding

For some, hoarding affords a sense of comfort and security. If your loved one is a hoarder and you find it poses a risk, you can address this by removing any dangerous items from their collection. Clutter, can also cause confusion and pose a risk.

You can try and negotiate by telling your loved one why the items you are removing are unsafe; however, negotiating with your loved one might not be realistic. Try to be as understanding and tactful as possible. I am sure you heard people say, "It's not so much what you say but how you say it." Your tone can convey more meaning than your actual words. At the end of the day, if negotiating isn't in the cards, just remove these items when they are out of their room. You need to be a little tricky because it's not worth an argument, and getting your loved one upset can do more harm than good. Oftentimes, they won't even miss the removed object(s). An empathy-driven emotional response will help to preserve your loved one's dignity without making them feel that they're mentally unfit or that they're being backed into a corner.

Shuffling Feet, Jittery Feet, and Unstable Gait

Shuffling feet while walking, including jittery feet, unstable gait, moving slowly, or standing in one place for an extended period of time, are all things that affect balance and can cause your loved one to fall repeatedly.

These behaviors can result from:

- Cognitive decline
- Loss of muscle coordination
- Dementia (in particular Lewy Body Dementia)
- Medication side effects
- Unregulated blood sugar levels (diabetics)

If your loved one is experiencing any of these behaviors, you can consult with a physical therapist and their doctor to see if medications or blood sugar levels need to be addressed and to add on exercises and activities to improve muscle coordination and reduce cognitive decline.

Changes in Eating and Drinking Habits and Abilities

Drastic shifts in eating habits might occur where your loved one will have a diminished appetite, not feel like eating, or desire to eat something that is not available. You might find that your loved one's taste buds have done a 180; foods and flavors that they did enjoy are now disliked. Food and flavors that they disliked may become favorites.

In this new world, anything is possible. Their new food choices might not align with prior beliefs and preferences. A person who's been a lifelong vegetarian may want to eat meat because they've forgotten they don't eat meat. They may see someone eating meat and decide they want to try it, or if their long-term memory kicks in, they might remember eating meat and not remember becoming a vegetarian.

Another example can be shared by telling the story of Sylvia, who, being of the Jewish persuasion, kept a Kosher home. She would never consider bringing any type of non-Kosher meat (pork) or shellfish into her home. She would never mix meat and cheese - so chicken parmesan was a no-no. Sylvia only wanted to eat shrimp, lobster, and bacon cheeseburgers, which her family knew she would never have eaten. However, her family came to realize that it no longer was an issue to her, or added any meaningful value to her. I know it was harder for Sylvia's family, for Sylvia had no remembrance or understanding of what Kosher was.

If your loved one insists on only eating sweet foods, do your best to provide healthier options. Sweet foods, fruits, and veggies are better options than processed foods like candy and cake. Adding small amounts of jam, honey, or syrup to food can increase the sweetness without taking a toll on blood sugar levels and can simultaneously satiate a sweet tooth.

In addition, there may come a time when your loved one may not be able to understand what they're putting into their mouth - soap, batteries, napkins, keys, and buttons are all possibilities. Make sure that you keep a sharp eye on, or keep any of these potential swallowing/choking hazards out of their reach. As the disease progresses, there might come a time when your loved one no longer remembers how to chew and swallow, and pureed food or liquid drinks become their only option for nutrition. With the progression of the disease, your loved one may even develop issues with drinking water, whereby you may need to introduce thickeners to avoid the possibility of choking. Straws have also been found to be detrimental in this regard.

Incontinence

As brain function declines, so does the frequency and accuracy of the messages going between the brain and the bladder or bowel. Your loved one may not understand that they have a full bladder or bowel, and they may not be able to control their bathroom urges.

In the early to mid stage of dementia, your doctor can intervene and help you with your loved one's incontinence issues and, in addition, can pinpoint underlying conditions that might contribute to the incontinence. These conditions can include UTI, constipation, dietary problems, or medicinal side effects.

If incontinence remains an issue, despite your and your doctor's efforts, there are many incontinence aids available.

These aids include pads, adult diapers, male incontinence sheaths, waterproof mattress protectors, absorbent bed pads, etc. All of these aids can be helpful in keeping your loved one comfortable while protecting their clothing, mattress, and other bedding. If your loved one is not yet exhibiting signs of incontinence and they are mobile, they may have trouble finding their way to the bathroom at night. My suggestion is for you to have a commode that you can keep near their bed, somewhere in their eye-line, so that they do not have to endure the challenge of getting to the bathroom in time. Ensure that there is adequate lighting (night lights) in both the bedroom and bathroom. Another helpful hint is to eliminate or reduce liquids after dinner.

Mobility Difficulties

More often than not, elder patients struggle with some degree of age-related mobility issues. When your loved one has dementia, related mobility issues are compounded. This is a result of the effect the disease has on the various parts of the brain, which are responsible for balance and muscle coordination. Mobility issues pose several challenges, such as an unsteady gait and an increased potential for losing balance and falling, and as the disease progresses, it may become difficult for your loved one to get in or out of bed independently. The ability and effort required to shift from sitting to standing or even lying down can become a struggle. In more severe cases, as the disease progresses to its final stage, complete immobility can occur.

To help your loved one manage the various mobility issues while they're in the early to mid stage, you can arrange to have mobility aids on hand. Such aids include: walkers, canes, and wheelchairs. Stability has never been more important, so choose shoes that have non-slip soles, which will help your loved one retain better balance.

If your goal, is to try and delay the progression of immobility, there are basic balancing exercises and mild muscle strengthening exercises, which will help your loved one keep their muscles limber, as well as help them to maintain their balance.

None of these exercises should be too arduous, and you can determine how much or how little your loved one can handle.

In addition to dementia affecting your loved one's mobility, it also will affect their senses, judgment, sense of time and place, behavior, and physical ability. Therefore, it is essential that you create an environment that will ensure their safety. This is so important, that I have provided you with more detailed information in Chapter 11, including multiple tips to ensure your success.

Personal Hygiene or Lack Thereof

Throughout the stages of dementia, your loved one will require varying levels of assistance from you. It's common for people with dementia to neglect their personal hygiene. They might find themselves unable to perform simple tasks or may simply lose interest and not care about maintaining good personal hygiene - bathing, shaving, clipping their nails, brushing their teeth, washing their face and hands, and changing their clothes.

As their caregiver, you will have the responsibility of ensuring that they maintain good personal hygiene. Don't worry; I have provided tips to help you with these issues:

Bathing / Showering

Get ready for a fight because oftentimes, you will get resistance from your loved one when it's time to get bathed. They may be uncomfortable or shy about having to have someone do for them what they used to do for themselves. If you can provide them with some privacy, by pulling down blinds and closing curtains and doors, this could minimize their self-consciousness. You want to allow your loved one to maintain their dignity, and these simple tips can go a long way. If your loved one no longer recognizes themself, you may simply cover or remove mirrors. You can make the bathroom more inviting by creating a comfortable temperature and welcoming environment (like a day at the spa). This can be accomplished with lighting, soft music, etc.

If your loved one gives you a hard time, the best thing you can do is to try and make it quick - rinse, wash, dry, and done (or cut the steps by using cleaning products that don't require any water.) At some point, you might need to modify the tub/shower to have room for a bench for sitting, a walker, or a wheelchair. At this point, you may need assistance because this can easily become a two-person job. As always, put safety first. If it gets to the point where you can no longer get your loved one into the bathroom for their shower/bath, they can stay in the comfort of their own bed and have a sponge bath. Likewise, they can have their hair washed with dry shampoo.

Shaving

An electric razor is recommended instead of a traditional/straight razor. Your loved one may be able to use this on their own; in some cases, it might give them a feeling of independence. If a straight razor shave is still important to your loved one, and if it is not safe for them to use a straight razor, you can take your loved one to a barber shop, which could turn into a fun outing, or you can arrange for someone to come to the house.

Oral Hygiene

In the early stage of dementia, your loved one may simply need a reminder to wash up and brush their teeth, but as the disease progresses, odds are you will need to do this for them. I would recommend switching to a soft toothbrush and using mild mouthwash instead of using something pungent and bitter. I would further suggest flossing, but make sure that you use a gentle floss or water pick so that you don't have to deal with bleeding gums.

Nail Care

It is important that your loved one's nails are cut and maintained as needed, as this can lead to cuts, infections, etc. If necessary, you can enlist the services of a podiatrist, who will deal with all foot-related issues and will even cut your loved one's nails if you are uncomfortable doing so. For a fun activity, if able, you can again take your loved one for an outing to the nail salon, where they can enjoy a manicure & pedicure.

Hair Care

Hair care can become a pleasure (or not). If you are able to take your loved one to a salon or barber, that too can become a special outing, and if that is not possible, there are stylists who will come to your home. Oftentimes, your loved one will enjoy a visit from the hairdresser or barber.

If and when you feel you need help, seek it out. There are professional healthcare and social workers who have experience in dealing with these issues and can provide you with further insight and ways to help you tackle these challenges.

Now, let's jump into a really tough topic: addressing whether or not you need to consider placing your loved one in an outside care facility.

Chapter 7

At Home Care or Outside Care Facility - What's Best for You and Your Loved One

Sometimes, you have to break a promise; that you swore you never would. There are times when with the best intentions, caregivers have promised their loved one that they would NEVER put them into an outside care facility and that no matter what the circumstance, they would be able to live in their home or yours forever.

When these promises were made, there is no doubt in the promiser's mind that their promise was forever. When making such a promise, it was without understanding or imagining what dementia could mean, or what it would be like to live with someone battling this disease, or be responsible for providing the necessary care. I have a story to share with you, that can offer a realistic perspective.

Nancy Helton, was the regional director of operations for Superior Residences, a memory-care assisted-living facility in Ocala, Florida. She said, "Every caregiver who comes to my desk, having promised their loved one that they would never do this, is fearful, saddened, and worst of all, feeling tremendous guilt."

Here, I am going to build upon Nancy's statement by telling you that the other typically displayed emotion is caused by the stigma surrounding the entire issue. It is painful for families who have made this promise to realize that they are left with no choice but to seek placement in an outside care facility. This decision can be agonizing, as well as, create a new sense of defeat and hopelessness.

With all your love and best intentions, you must understand that there could come a time, for a variety of reasons, that you no longer can fulfill your promise, regardless of the sacrifices you are willing to make. Sometimes, through no fault of your own, the decision is no longer a possible one to avoid. My goal is that you, my reader, have the information, tools, and assistance, in order for you to make the best decision for your loved one - whether it is for you to be the primary caregiver, hire an in-home caregiver, or need to consider an outside care facility.

Throughout this chapter, I will paint you a picture of the various options available to consider, so that you can decide what the best choice would be for you and your loved one.

If finances allow or if you already have a home health care policy in place, you can hire a person or people to assist you in providing care for your loved one at home.

Home Care Options

Outside homecare service providers, offer you the caregiver professional assistance within the home. This can be provided by an independent caregiver, who can be hired as an independent contractor, or can be provided by professional homecare agencies that train and employ professional caregivers. These caregivers can provide daily care assistance (cooking, bathing, hygiene care, etc.), dementia care and supervision, and companionship. These services can be provided contractually or paid hourly.

Home care comes in different forms. If necessary, consult with your doctor or a healthcare professional to determine the type of home healthcare that would be best suited for your loved one. Most importantly, consider your own personal needs and assistance desires.

A main advantage of choosing at-home care is that your loved one can remain in their familiar surroundings, which, for a person with dementia, can be soothing and create a more relaxed environment.

Another advantage, equally as important, for in-home support, is for you, the primary caregiver. Having this assistance, if only for a few hours, can afford you the opportunity to have time for yourself. Relax, get together with friends, do errands, take a drive, or simply have a drink and unwind.

While these caregivers are equipped to handle your loved one's day-to-day care, they aren't equipped to provide skilled nursing care.

They can offer the following services:

- **Transportation** - from home to the hospital, doctor's office visits, and other desired outings.

- **Every Day Tasks** - meal preparation, assistance eating, drinking, or homemaking tasks, including cleaning, laundry, bedding, etc.
- **Companionship** - this can range from a few hours every day to 24-hour care, if needed. Dementia patients require companionship; as the primary caregiver, you may have to work, which may preclude you from being able to provide 24/7 care. You will want to have someone available to provide this companionship, whether it's simply to have a conversation with, look through picture books, or watch TV. The key to this, is to provide some form of stimulation for your loved one and not have them sit in a chair or lay in a bed doing nothing all day. The more your loved one is engaged, the better it will be for them.
- **Personal Care -** Depending upon the level of personal care required, which can include getting dressed, bathroom needs, personal hygiene, bathing, wound care, diaper change, etc., you will be able to determine the degree of care necessary. Around-the-clock care, will most probably become needed when dealing with the later stages of dementia.
- **Dementia Care** - helping with behavioral issues, including anxiety, frustration, wandering, etc.
- **Respite Care** - Respite care can serve as a temporary relief for you, the primary caregiver. These services will range in duration depending upon your need. This care can range from a few hours, to a week, or longer. You may be under the weather, need to go out of town (wedding, funeral, getting your kid settled in at college, etc.), or you may just need a break and

take that much-needed and deserved vacation. Respite care can make your life as the primary caregiver more livable.

- **Home Health Care / Nursing Care -** If skilled medical care becomes a necessity, there are options for home health care, that include hiring a nurse. Nursing care is specialized and is a considerably more expensive option, for your loved one who may require a higher degree of care. In this case, a home nursing professional would come to your home and administer such medical care as: examining the patient, dressing wounds if necessary, administering any injectable medications, and reviewing current drug doses, while discussing any new concerns or observances you, the caregiver, may have come upon. These nurses will work with you to establish ongoing care and help you redesign routines, if necessary, to meet your loved one's ever-changing needs. Any of the nurse's findings, should be shared and discussed with your loved one's physician, and they should be in agreement as to ongoing care and related changes.

If the time has come and it becomes necessary to seek alternatives, other than at-home care, you should become familiar with the various types of options available, as well as, understand what your loved one's caregiving currently requires.

Care Facility Options

Memory Care Facilities

Memory care facilities are specifically designed to cater to patients with dementia and are usually a specialized area within a larger elder care facility. Here, trained professionals and nurses are available to care for patients throughout their varying stages of dementia.

These facilities provide your loved one with care designed to improve their quality of life by reducing stimulation and disorientation through secure settings with on-site professionals.

These facilities provide all the services offered in traditional assisted living facilities, such as medication management, daily living assistance, meal preparation, etc. In addition, they provide specific amenities catering to patients with cognitive disabilities.

In these facilities, patients are monitored by a professional 24/7. Safety features are ensured and include security cameras, locked doors, emergency call buttons, orderlies monitoring the corridors, etc. The living spaces are designed in such a way to make the patient feel "at home" and feel comfortable, and safe. Examples of this would include: walls painted in soothing colors, hallways clearly lit and designed so that patients can wander without fear of injury, a personalized picture or object to identify one's room, and colors or pictures associated with a specific activity. Having this comfortable living space can reduce depression, anxiety, and agitation. If a patient does tend to wander, there are hallways and layouts, that allow them to wander without feeling trapped or worried about getting lost. Often, there are also multisensory rooms for therapy and relaxation. Most facilities have outside areas designed with safe, calming gardens and courtyards for the patient to walk in (or be wheeled in), interact with, and explore. The staff should be trained in behavioral interventions that can mitigate symptoms such as hallucinations, disorientation, aggression, etc., when they are exhibited.

Several types of supportive therapies and activities take place in memory care facilities. These can include pet therapy, massage therapy, art therapy, music therapy, sensory therapy, reminiscence therapy, etc. - the list is endless. Programs and activities are also provided in order to provide companionship and promote social interaction, as both are essential elements that can enhance their quality of life and reduce feelings of aggression and isolation.

Nursing Homes

A nursing home is a facility that provides residential and healthcare accommodations. There are some nursing homes that specifically provide care for persons with dementia, within their facility; however, you want to be sure that the facility you choose, has this dedicated unit, which could be a floor or a building, but that specifically caters to patients with dementia. In such a facility, you can have assurance that the staff has expertise in this area. Be sure to do your research and confirm that the nursing home takes on full custodial care, whereby their staff ensures their patients have everything and anything necessary for their care, safety, and well-being.

Another important consideration, is the nursing home's policy on how they handle hospital visits. Does the facility care for their sick patient in-house until a hospital becomes absolutely necessary, or do they send them to the hospital at the first sign of illness? In addition, you will want to know the facility's policy on hospital discharge. Does the patient automatically go back to the nursing home, or does the nursing home have discretion on whether or not to accept the patient back? You also want to know if there are in-house physicians, if not, do physicians visit the facility, or do patients get transported back and forth to the doctor's office? If so, who from the facility goes with them? These questions should also be asked in regard to dentists. Do dentists come in regularly, are their in-house dentists, or, again, does the patient need to go to the dentist's office?

Group Home

Another consideration, would be a private group home, licensed and set up to care for dementia patients. In this environment, the patient is living in someone's home (with a living room, kitchen, and all home amenities) that has been converted into a care facility. This environment may be a good option because it puts your loved one into a more familiar environment and can sometimes provide a more home-like and personal experience, whereby other patients become like friends or family, and they are apt to find the socialization and personal touches, that are so important.

Assisted Living

Another type of facility, known as assisted living, is for people who choose to be in an environment with other people either because they no longer want to live by themselves or no longer can care for themselves 100%, but are basically able to function without individualized assistance. Unfortunately, this would not be a long-term option for your loved one with dementia and, therefore, not a viable option.

As this can be an extremely overwhelming choice, there are many options and things to consider before making this decision.

Things to Consider When Choosing a Care Facility

Cost/Financial ability - financial where-with-all, in-place care insurance policies, state and/or federal assistance, etc.

Proximity to your home or other family members - It is important to consider the proximity to your home so that you can visit often.

It is important to find a facility that has a **specialized department for dementia patients.**

When you visit, be sure to: choose different times of the day to visit facilities, visit the dining room during mealtimes, review menu choices, and visit and talk with the staff there as well as other patients and their family members who are visiting. Observe how the residents look specifically as to grooming and care.

Be sure to inquire as to their "open door policy." You will want to know if you are welcome to visit anytime, walk the premises, have a meal with your loved one, and inquire as to accommodations regarding dietary restrictions.

If you are living in the US, ask to see the facility's state survey inspection report. If you are residing in the UK, ask for a copy of the Care Quality Commission (CQC) report. If you are in another country, check that country's equivalent.

You will want to determine whether the facility you choose can remain as a forever home. Once your loved one is living at the care facility, will they be able to remain there? You will want to make sure it is a facility that is capable of caring for your loved one through all stages of the disease, and if your loved one should run out of money, will they be able to remain living there?

Suggested Questions to Ask When Visting a Facility:

1. How does the facility ensure nutritious meals and that the food is eaten?
2. How do they handle specific dietary requirements?
3. Can the family join the patient for meals?
4. How does the facility communicate health and other issues to the family?
5. Does the facility notify the family when making alterations to their care plans?
6. What specific medical and personal care is provided on-site?
7. Is laundry service provided? Who determines when cleaning/laundering is necessary?

8. Are pets allowed (to live or visit)?
9. Is there a barber or beautician on-site or that comes to the facility regularly?
10. What is the ratio of nurses to patients? Is there always a registered nurse on the premises?
11. How often is a physician there, and how often will they see your loved one?
12. Does the facility take residents to medical appointments when needed?
13. What is the level of training regarding behavioral issues, and how are they handled?
14. How does the facility handle ER visits? Who accompanies the patient to the hospital? Will I immediately be contacted?
15. If desired, will my loved one have a home for life? What is the discharge policy? Is there any situation that would prompt the facility to discharge the patient, and if so, how much notice would you receive?
16. Is the facility equipped to handle hospice patients, or are they sent off-site?
17. Are religious services available - do they provide in-house services and bring in priests, rabbis, etc?
18. What types of entertainment and activities are provided?

Chapter 8
Hospice

Hospice

You will want to know what to expect if and when hospice becomes necessary. As dementia progresses and approaches its final stages, hospice may be an alternative you will need to seriously consider. Hospice is the final stop, as hospice provides comfort and dignity at the end of your loved one's life.

Perhaps that's why the mere mention of the word "hospice" is scary. Hospice and palliative care are synonymous. Once you agree to hospice care, whether in your home or a facility, all drugs other than those needed to avoid pain and discomfort are discontinued. Bringing your loved one to a hospital, once in hospice care, is no longer an option, as doing so will automatically terminate this care. Hospice is another horribly difficult decision to come to terms with. There are some major considerations you need to contemplate in order to make this important decision. Before we get ahead of ourselves, it is necessary for you to understand exactly what hospice care is.

Hospice Care's primary goal, is to focus on comfort rather than cure. End-stage dementia is considered to be a terminal illness, and hospice provides care and pain management during the final days and weeks of life. Hospice Care is usually considered, when a patient's life expectancy is six months or less. Your doctor should help you determine whether or not he or she feels your loved one is a candidate for this care. The hospice team is comprised of trained providers, including doctors, nurses, health care aides, social workers, clergy, counselors, and volunteers. The family can also be involved with hospice care, especially when the hospice care is done at home.

If your loved one is at home, you will be assigned a dedicated nurse(s) who will come to your home on a regular basis. They will determine how often you are visited (usually one to two times per week, or in some cases more often). They will check with you or your privately hired caregiver and examine your loved one, take their vitals, and review all medications to determine whether or not refills or changes are necessary. You will have an opportunity to discuss any changes or newly developed challenges in your loved one's care, since their last visit. They will be coordinating with the hospice doctor assigned to your loved one's case. You can reach out to your hospice nurse at any time and/or request a non-scheduled visit.

In addition to medications to keep your loved one comfortable, Hospice provides counseling and grief support for you, the caregiver, and other family members to help you confront this harsh emotional reality and help you prepare for it. Hospice professionals will be available to you and other family members of your loved one for as many months, up to a year, to provide you with grief counseling and suggestions for outside therapy to process your loss.

Hospice also provides resources to assist dementia patients on their spiritual journey. These resources are coordinated with the help of therapists, spiritualists, clergy, and religious figures, if desired. This assistance is meant to help the patient or family come to terms and can be very meaningful when coming to the realization that the end of the journey is approaching.

Moving forward, I will help you to hone and master your caregiving skills so that you have the proper tools to provide the most comfortable and safe environment, as your loved one continues in their cognitive decline.

In future chapters, I will go into greater detail to help you manage and understand the available insurance and legal matters. Although the contents of my book may prove emotionally challenging, my hope is that it will help you to understand the disease better, equip you with knowledge, and hopefully make this difficult situation less painful - remember you are not alone. One of my main desires in writing this book is to provide you and your loved one with empathetic care, while simultaneously giving you the support necessary to take care of yourself. Always remember that for you to be a good caregiver, you must stay healthy and do your best to give yourself T.L.C.

Chapter 9
Support and Tips Throughout Your Journey

When caring for a loved one with dementia, you're undertaking a journey that requires a great deal of patience, understanding, and awareness. Knowing what lies ahead and the reality of how the journey progresses is necessary and one that you must come to terms with. Although this is a difficult journey, the understanding and foresight you will hopefully glean from reading this book will make your journey as stress-free as possible. This disease can go on for a very long time (years). It can be tiring, stressful, and emotionally exhausting. Remember, this is not a sprint but a marathon. What makes this even more difficult, is that you are doing a thankless job, as you cannot expect any thank yous or signs of appreciation. This is why choosing to be the primary caregiver for your loved one is the most sincere expression of love and caring. The sacrifices you will undoubtedly be forced to make along the way, will make a huge difference in your loved one's quality of life, and you should remember it is the greatest gift you could ever give.

Although I have already painted the picture that caregiving is an all-consuming job, this only grows more and more intense as your loved one's dementia progresses with each passing stage. As your loved one's caregiver, you are the one who will witness firsthand their cognitive, functional, and physical decline. This emotional toll can pose health risks to you, which can include depression, stress, sadness, loneliness, anxiety, exhaustion, and, ultimately, burnout. Seeking help is so very important - it is a necessity, not a luxury.

In this chapter, I will provide you with the framework that should assist you on your caregiving journey. Although every caregiver's experience (just as a dementia patient's experience) is different, there are some general strategies that can help turn your caregiving journey into a rewarding experience. That's not to say there won't be challenges along the way - there most definitely will be. But through a structured approach, which is my objective to provide you with, there will also be many rewards.

If you're just beginning your caregiving journey, there are strategies that will be extremely helpful and beneficial for you to implement in the daily care you will provide to your loved one. Even early on in dementia, your loved one will experience remarkable changes in thinking, recalling things, and reasoning. While in the beginning, it won't affect their lives as drastically as later on, it will still have an impact on how they lead their daily life and how they perform their prior activities. They will require more assistance with daily tasks such as grooming, bathing, dressing, going for a walk, eating their food, going to the bathroom, etc.

For someone who hasn't experienced being a caregiver at such a personal level, some elements of this calling, can become extremely upsetting to both you, the caregiver, and your loved one.

Establishing and keeping a daily routine can significantly help to keep these emotions in check and make the journey as pleasant as possible for both you and your loved one.

Tips to Support Your Daily Routine

Get Organized

The first thing you should do, is create a calendar or planner to set up reminders for such things as personal hygiene, activities, and appointments, especially doctor appointments. I would suggest a simple calendar; however, any device you choose can be utilized. If your loved one is in the earlier stages, they may be capable, with or without your assistance, to share in entering their appointments or special time-related activities. A large calendar that can be placed on a kitchen counter or hung on the wall, works well (**LINK**). There are also calendars available that are divided into two halves. One half for the calendar itself and the other for pictures. This is especially nice to do, if you are hanging the calendar because the upside is always visible. On this portion of the calendar, you can have a picture of your choice, which in itself can become a memory activity. For example, if November is your loved one's son's birthday, you can choose a picture of him. There are tons of companies that make custom calendars. Just google personalized calendars, and you will find a large selection of options to choose from. However, if you are the sole user, your options are greater, as you can use your phone, computer, or any calendar app for this purpose. This is a good tool, so you do not have to overburden your memory with this information. As a caregiver, you will need to reserve that brilliant head of yours and not overload it with things that are unnecessary. At this stage, you will want to conserve your abilities and make things as simple and as easy as possible. As far as reminders for your loved one for things such as brushing teeth, bathing, mealtimes, etc., you can do something like this: on a piece of paper, you can create a "to-do" list for your loved one, i.e.: good morning, remember to brush your teeth and wash your face.... almost time to go to sleep, make sure you brush your teeth and wash your hands and face, etc.

Set Reminders

If your loved one is still in the earlier stages of the disease, they may be able to take their medications on their own, and if so, you want to have a reminder for them so that they know what to take and what time to take it. Even if your loved one is still able to handle this task, I strongly urge you to keep the medication bottles out of sight and use a weekly pill organizer so that all your loved one has to do, is open the appropriate day to take their medicine. They come in all shapes, colors, and sizes. Some split morning, noon, and night doses, and some even have auditory and visual reminder alarms. More than likely, you will be with them to assist, or in later stages, when you are administering their medications, it will be easier for you to follow the same suggestion by using a pill box to organize their daily meds.

Buy Clothing That is Both Comfortable and Easy to Get In and Out of and Wash

When dressing, depending upon your loved one's ability, they might be able to choose their own clothing for the day. Just as with all other activities, you need to decide if your loved one is up to the task, or if not, you can just have the clothing laid out for them to put on. If you are lying out their clothing, get them involved. Encourage them to have a say in what they would like to wear and offer them a choice. Here are some useful tips:

- Loose-fitting
- Breathable fabrics for clothing
- Opt for elastic waistbands
- Use zippers or fasteners as opposed to buttons, buckles, and laces
- Durable materials that are machine washable

Buy an Eyeglass Retainer

It's common for people with dementia to forget they wear glasses, no less keep track of them. Save yourself the hours of frustration you would otherwise spend throughout the day, looking for misplaced glasses. There is a fix! There are many choices when purchasing eyewear retainers, commonly known as eyeglass lanyards or straps. These simply hook onto the arms of the glasses and stay around your loved one's neck just as would a necklace.

Tips for Maintaining a Healthy Lifestyle (these are tips for both you and your loved one)

Healthy Diet

A healthy diet tops the list of important lifestyle changes. An appropriately active lifestyle for your loved one and an active lifestyle for yourself are both extremely important. In the later stage of dementia, when eating healthy food becomes an issue, getting them to eat can become very challenging; no less, getting them to eat their greens.

Now, it's time to get creative. Try your best, not to make them feel like you are forcing them to eat something, or to engage in an activity that they don't seem to be comfortable with. Rather, consider substituting another food you know they like together with the food you are trying to get them to eat, i.e.: they love spaghetti with red sauce but are not interested in any protein, you can grind up sausages or meatballs into the sauce, so they won't be able to tell that meat is incorporated into the dish. As far as activities, try to engage them in those activities they appear to enjoy. For instance, tell them you need help baking or cooking and then find a recipe that is appropriate. You do the measuring, they do the pouring, you mix, then hand them the bowl to continue the mixing.

As a matter of fact, another one of my patients, Sally, told me that her mother was sitting in her wheelchair at the kitchen table, while she was busy cooking and baking. Sally went over to her mother and told her she couldn't get everything done in time and asked for her help making the dessert. She gave her mother a bowl and three measuring cups (plastic), making sure that none of them were too full or heavy, and had her mom pour the ingredients into the measuring cups. Then, one by one, she had her mother pour the ingredients into a bowl with a pour spout and stir. She told me her mother had so much fun, and she was delighted to see her mom with a smile on her face. Although Sally helped and supervised, to ensure that the end product would be edible, she actually didn't care because it provided a wonderful adventure for her mom. Sally, cooking by the oven, just steps away from her mom, watched as her mom was very busy mixing and stirring. She was delighted to see that after just a few minutes, her mom began to hum and was truly engaging in this activity. When Sally noticed her mom was done, she gave her mother a pan and held it while supervising her mom as she poured the mixture into the pan. Her mom watched as Sally put the pan into the oven. Sally purposely put the timer on for 50 minutes, so that her mom could hear the timer go off. Her mother did not want to leave the kitchen because she wanted to hear the timer go off, humming the whole time. When the timer went off, Sally opened the oven, turned to her mother, and said: "Boy, this smells delicious. I hope it tastes as good as it smells." As Sally took the cake out of the oven, her mother was still smiling. After allowing it to cool, she brought it to the table and cut a slice for her and her mom to enjoy. Her mother had such a big smile as she devoured the piece of cake. Sally said that she took a bite and couldn't believe how delicious the cake tasted - she said it was the best cake she ever made. I wondered whether this was actually the best cake Sally ever made, or if it was just the fact that Sally's mother was so proud and happy to have participated in making the cake, that made it taste so extra wonderfully delicious to Sally. This positive experience gave Sally the idea to turn this into a shared project in the days, weeks, and months to follow. Sally discovered that an added bonus to her spending such enjoyable time with her mom, was that her mom was also excited to eat the food she so enjoyed making. If you decide to make this a shared experience for you and your loved one, be sure to take advantage and use ingredients that are healthy, easy to swallow, and digest.

Exercise

As far as exercise goes, instead of hectic workouts that are not feasible, consider taking your loved one on a short walk (or wheel them, if in a wheelchair) somewhere pretty and stop along the way to sit and people-watch, or simply just sit and talk. This will not only be beneficial to your loved one but will be beneficial to you as well.

Most people with dementia either have trouble or have little or no desire to engage in physical activities, nor do they stay motivated when engaged. Oftentimes, if you join them in the activity, they will be more inclined to participate and stay involved.

Tips to Take Care of YOUR Mental Health

Take Breaks When Needed

To prevent you from exhaustion, feeling socially isolated, angry, or frustrated, it is imperative that you take regular breaks and shift your focus from your loved one to yourself. If you have the ability to bring in outside help, or can call upon a friend or family member, don't be shy about asking for assistance. If you do not have the financial wherewithal to hire someone and do not have a willing family member or friend, you can look to your house of worship or other local community organizations, where volunteers may be available to be called upon.

Create or Join a Support Group

Support groups are available, whether they're online or in person. Besides providing actual assistance in your home, you can also use such groups to connect with other caregivers who may be able to share ideas and experiences that you have not dealt with, or thought of. Sometimes, just talking to someone who is going, or has gone through, the same experience that you are, can be extremely comforting. You can make a new friend and have someone to talk to who totally understands what you are going through. Remember the saying, misery loves company? That might sound like a cliche, but sometimes it is very true. Just knowing someone is walking in your shoes, and going through a similar situation helps you to feel that you are not on an island, and that you are not alone. You can also exchange some valuable pointers to help each other become better caregivers. I have created a Facebook group you can join by using this link: https://www.facebook.com/groups/272377975780751, or by scanning the QR code below.

I welcome you to become part of this community, as having a trusted friend or family member who appreciates your perspective, listens to you, judgment-free, can provide you with valuable insight, from their own experiences. This can result in a catharsis and act as a stress reliever.

Take Some Time to do the Things You Enjoy

What is your jam? Meditation? Exercise? Playing video games? Reading a book? Watching TV? Catching up on social media? Spend time engaging in your favorite hobbies. These are all activities that can give you the daily break you need to recharge for the rest of the day. You can invite a friend over and have a cup of coffee (or wine) with them.

Janice, a friend from childhood, told me that a gal she knew from the neighborhood, came home from college to visit her family. During her visit, Janice invited her friend to her house and Janice's mother came into the room to join them. Although not being sure who this neighbor was, Janice's mom believed her to be "her" old friend and thought she was there for a long overdue visit.

On a more personal level, I have a story to share. After my dad's divorce, he started dating his prior high school sweetheart, Randy, who was my grandmother's best friend's daughter. When they became seriously involved, he started visiting and was reintroduced to her mom, who suffered from dementia. Randy's mom was convinced that my dad was her old boyfriend - not Randy's boyfriend. My dad was kind enough to play along. This experience made Randy's mom feel special and important, and also allowed for some levity to an otherwise sad situation. P.S. Randy is now my step-mom, and my father was able to share Randy's caregiving experience and was instrumental in providing much-needed care to her, by assisting her not only with responsibilities but also providing relief and much-needed companionship during this trying period.

Tips for Dealing With the Initial Diagnosis of Dementia and the Corresponding Grief

When your loved one is initially diagnosed with dementia, processing the news together will help in coming to terms and acceptance. Try to include your loved one when planning for the future, as well as do your best to keep them active and engaged. Yes, this can also be a time to grieve. If your loved one is sad and appears to be grieving, allow them this time and space to process their emotions and grieve alongside them. Grief is a natural step in processing loss and paves the way for acceptance. If you try to ignore it altogether, it can cause denial to prevail and can also inhibit early intervention.

Grief is only one of the conflicting emotions that you and your loved one will experience. Other emotions include: anger, regret, denial, frustration, sadness, depression, confusion, and hostility. Just as the disease progresses, these conflicting emotions progress as well. Encourage your loved one to confide in you and allow them to express themselves and share their feelings.

Although we already spoke about community-based and online resources, an Alzheimer's / Dementia association in your area will have a plethora of resources available, such as: training, helplines, practical support, etc., which you should avail yourself of, as much as possible. Any advice and information you are able to obtain, will be a great source to help you in your caregiving role.

Tips on How to Mitigate Life Changes Associated with Independence

As the disease progresses, there will be more and more reasons that your loved one will feel a loss of independence, as well as, require more care and assistance. At this stage, you might feel that you need additional support in your role as primary caregiver. Your loved one will begin or continue to experience more pronounced memory loss, causing them to feel lost - even in their own home. They should not be driving any longer, and this can be an incredibly difficult concept for them to understand and again, I am here to help.

Here are some tips that will better enable you to approach the "taking the keys away" conversation:

- Time to get creative - **find excuses** for them not to drive. These can include: (1) The car needs repairs before it can be driven safely, i.e.: it needs a new battery, and the mechanic won't arrive until later this week. (2) Express concerns about weather conditions, traffic, or road safety (3) Come up with a legal reason for them not to be able to drive, i.e.: expired tags or license, etc. By employing some of these creative excuses, the restriction becomes way less personal. Blame the DMV for not allowing them to drive. Explain that the DMV will not renew their license.
- **Distract and redirect their focus** - if you sense an argument that is about to ensue, think quickly and try to switch the subject, hoping that they won't remember why they were getting upset, or the subject of their anger. "Your glasses are all dirty," and offer to clean them. "You won't believe what I found hidden in

the garage; I have to show you these photos" (or another item to grab their attention). Before they can respond to the initial detractor, suggest an alternate activity to distract them further. Asking for help with small tasks makes them feel needed and empowered, i.e.: drawer that won't close or need help finding something.

- **Reassure them -** in any situation where your loved one is feeling uncomfortable, whether it's having had to give up the keys to their car, or cooking their own meals, it makes no difference. The way to avoid this and make sure that your loved one never experiences these feelings of fear associated with loss of independence, is to offer them reassurance. Reassure them that you will always be there for them. They will always have someone with them to take them wherever they need or want to go (within reason).
- **Remember to be kind to yourself** - do not harbor feelings of guilt. If you believe the time has come for them to stop driving and that they are no longer safe to get behind the wheel, trust your judgment. There is a reason; trust your instincts. Taking the keys at the appropriate time, alleviates the risk of them harming themselves, or others, and most likely will save you, the caregiver, from having a nervous breakdown.

Tips for Late Stage Dementia

As your loved one reaches the end stage of dementia, more extensive care will be required. Twenty-four-hour care, may now be necessary. Your loved one may no longer be able to walk or sit/rise safely without assistance. Difficulties can occur when eating, going to the bathroom, communicating, etc. At this time infections, incontinence, hallucinations, delirium, mood swings, and everything else under the sun will increase and must be addressed. Aside from caregiving, an important role as caregiver, will be to preserve your loved one's dignity and quality of life. Tips to assist:

- **Food and fluids must be monitored,** so ensure your loved one is drinking enough fluids to prevent dehydration. Ensure your loved one is consuming and/or eating, i.e.: Ensure, Glucerna, etc., to prevent malnutrition and unsafe weight loss. Foods will need to be tailored to accommodate both health and safety restrictions, i.e.: softer foods, chopped, pureed foods, and liquids (which may require thickening). It is important that your loved one be able to swallow without it becoming a potential choking hazard.
- **Ensure that eating and drinking are done in an upright position,** and it is suggested that they remain in this position for thirty minutes after eating or drinking to allow for better digestion.
- If **incontinence** becomes an ongoing challenge during late-stage of dementia, be sure you are well stocked with incontinence products such as: adult disposable briefs and diapers and absorbent and protective sheets. Limit liquids before bedtime in the evening (after dinner).
- **Monitor bowel movements** and if they are constipated or have diarrhea, treat them accordingly.
- If your loved one is bedridden, be sure to keep creams and products on hand to **prevent skin breakdown, pressure sores, joint freezing**, etc. It is

important to prevent bedsores, so aside from massaging and creaming, turn your loved one regularly, every two hours, or so, to relieve body pressure and improve blood circulation. Use pillows to prop their arms and legs and ensure that they're in a comfortable position. Padding bony areas can help to prevent injuries and rashes. Range-of-motion exercises can help to prevent joints from freezing.

- Knowing how to move and lift your loved one to **adjust their position** in bed and/or get them out of bed will ensure that they are not hurt in the process. A physical therapist or a licensed nurse will be able to teach you how this is done.
- An added tip to **prevent infections** would be to maintain healthy oral hygiene and treat all bruises and wounds immediately. Be sure to take protective measures in order to avoid common viruses, such as the flu and pneumonia, by keeping your loved one up to date on vaccinations.
- **Communication** will decline as the disease progresses. Be sure to pay attention to non-verbal cues and check for physical manifestations resulting from pain and illnesses. Examples can include: bleeding gums, pale skin, redness, bruising, or swelling of the body. During this time, you will need to be even more observant of changes in your loved one's behavior, which can be manifested by unprovoked agitation or trembling.
- **Utilizing assistive technology** such as baby monitors and in-home video monitors can be a great help in taking some of the stress off, because you can keep an eye on them when you are not able to be in

their room.

Chapter 10
Strategies to Manage Communication Challenges

Many changes occur with each passing stage of the disease. Communication is one area that is greatly affected throughout the disease. The level of contingency is based on the stage of the disease. As the disease continues to spiral, so does the deterioration of your loved one's communication.

To make this easier to understand, imagine that their brain is going back in time, just like in the movie, "The Curious Case of Benjamin Button," where Benjamin goes from old man to young adult, to teen, to adolescent, and so on. As this occurs, communication with your loved one will require continued patience, active listening, empathy, and ongoing understanding.

I want to again emphasize, that becoming impatient, angry, frustrated, and hostile towards your loved one is the worst form of communication and should be avoided at all costs.

I will provide you with some of the finer points of communicating with your loved one to facilitate better communication. This will vary based on the stage and rate at which their specific type of dementia progresses.

The specific changes in communication, which vary from the early, middle, and late stages of the disease, should be shared with your family members as well, so that they too, can have the best potential for success in communicating with your loved one, throughout each of these stages.

Early-Stage Communication

If the diagnosis has been recognized in the early stage, your loved one should still be able to take part in meaningful conversations, should still be able to recall many things, and, therefore, should be encouraged to continue their participation in social activities.

At some point, you will begin to recognize a decline in their mental capabilities. They will begin by repeating phrases, telling the same story over and over, and may become overwhelmed with stimulation. You will begin to notice a great reduction in both their vocabulary, and their struggle to find the right words, will become harder and harder.

Optimize communication during this period:

- Include your loved one in conversations. Take the time to listen to your loved one, allowing them the time to express themselves completely, before interrupting or interjecting with the right words.
- Allow your loved one ample time to respond - do not rush them.
- Create opportunities so that your loved one can make simple choices.

- When asking questions, make them simple and clear. If offering options, limit them to 1 or 2. Too many options, can become extremely confusing.
- Speak directly to your loved one and always have eye contact.
- Allow your loved one to be repetitive.
- Always use your loved one's name.
- Practice becoming a good listener (active listening techniques are useful) and listen carefully, not just to the words being said, as you should also observe your loved one's facial expressions and behavior.
- Avoid interruptions while conversing with your loved one and try to minimize distractions.
- Always encourage your loved one to engage in conversations and provide as many opportunities, as possible.
- Allow your loved one to speak for themselves, when spoken to.
- Rephrase questions when necessary.
- Redirect any negative words, by replacing them with a positive choice, as negativity yields negativity. For example: replace words such as no, do not, cannot, should not, with: let us do this first, wouldn't it be fun to, what if we, etc.
- Use a reassuring and comforting tone of voice and redirect your loved one by taking their attention off the situation that is causing their anxiety.
- Use positive action statements to get your loved one to engage in a desired activity, i.e.: Come with me, I love it when we have dinner together.

Middle-Stage (Moderate Dementia) Communication

This is the longest stage of the disease and can last several years. Your loved one will have more difficulty in communicating and will require more care, especially in terms of communication. You and your family members should:

- Speak in a slow and clear voice, enunciate your words - make sure your tone is not condescending.
- Engage your loved one in one-on-one conversations, in a quiet place without distractions.
- Maintain eye contact with your loved one, which provides them with the sense that you care about what they are saying.
- Be very patient with your loved one and offer affirmation and reassurance, which should encourage them to have a continued desire to express themselves.
- As in the earlier stage, continue to limit your questions - one at a time, and wait for a response, or repeat the question, as if you're asking it for the first time.
- When feasible, attempt to elicit questions that require only a yes or no response. Options and choices should be limited to a "this" or "that" response.
- Criticism of any kind is not helpful, nor is offering corrections.
- When giving instructions, do so one step at a time, using short, simple sentences.
- Never argue with your loved one. If they say something that you disagree with, just let it slide. There are no winners; become a "yes man."
- When possible, use visual cues to demonstrate a task.

- Remain fluid and flexible - follow Bruce Lee's well-known and expert advice, which is: "Be Water, My Friend."
- Smile, breathe, and relax—your calmness will become contagious and will both comfort your loved one and reduce any exhibited agitation.

Late-Stage Communication

In the late stage, also known as severe dementia, verbal communication will become extremely difficult, and your loved one will need to rely on non-verbal cues. These can include: vocal sounds, hand gestures, and facial expressions. I suggest:

- When approaching your loved one, you should always be facing them. Identify yourself by name and relation ("I'm your son, John" or "I'm your cousin, Clara.")
- If your loved one is experiencing difficulty with speech, encourage them to communicate through gestures.
- If hearing is impaired, consider purchasing a hearing device or aide (if you can get them to wear it), if not, try communicating in written or picture form.
- Utilize sounds, sights, smells, and tastes as forms of communication.
- Be creative - try and understand what you believe they are trying to communicate.
- If you are not achieving success, having tried the above suggestions, try a guessing game. Hold up different items and watch for any facial recognition, etc.

Chapter 11
Setting Your Home Up For Safety & Comfort

Home Safety

Dementia affects both the brain and bodily functions, which can affect your loved one in many ways, including their safety. Safety is such an important area of concern, that I deemed it necessary to highlight, by devoting an entire chapter to this issue. This disease will impact a multitude of your loved one's behaviors and senses. Your loved one may forget how to use common household equipment and appliances. Their sense of time and space can get warped, which can result in their getting lost in familiar neighborhood surroundings, or even in later stages, getting lost in their own home.

Physical challenges will arise and their ability to balance themselves can become even more pronounced. This can result in a trip or fall and can even be attributed to difficulty in getting up from, or into their bed or chair. The parts of the brain affected by dementia can also diminish one's senses, causing changes in their ability to hear, perceive depth, see, and taste, as well as, their sensitivity to varying temperatures. Accordingly, is vital to ensure that your home is a safe and secure environment.

Tips to Create a Dementia-Safe Environment

- Remove obstacles such as rugs and runners, or place non-slip pads if removal is not a possibility, to prevent potential tripping hazards.
- Avoid extension cords or secure cords to the floor or walls.
- Install rails for support in areas such as stairwells, shower/bath, and toilet.
- Make sure areas are well-lit and install lights where needed (night lights or motion-activated lights can be great options).
- Maintain and check to be sure that all smoke alarms and carbon monoxide alarms are in working order.
- Indicate heating vents, steps, stairwells, and any other potential dangers with red tape or caution stickers. Symbols or warning signs can remind a person with dementia of unsafe areas.
- Place decals on windows and doors or glass surfaces to avoid accidents.
- Place safety covers on all electrical outlets.
- Install child-proof safety locks on cabinets, drawers, doors, fridge, and any other appliances, as needed.
- Remove or secure any hazardous items, or at least be sure that they are out of reach.
- Remove glass tabletops and/or furniture with sharp corners when possible. Alternatively, there are

products available, such as corner protectors. There are many baby-proofing items readily available to minimize areas of danger. All of these suggestions can help to eliminate unnecessary accidents.

- Remove clutter, and by doing so can help to avoid tripping and falling.
- Non-skid pads available for chair legs can help to stabilize chairs.
- Avoid the use of electric blankets.
- Get rid of any poisonous plants from your collection.

Your **kitchen** has now become an area that requires your attention, when it comes to safety. Here are some tips to ensure that your kitchen can still be a favorite room to congregate:

- Make sure you have a fire extinguisher, and it is easily within your reach.
- Install an anti-scald device for the sink to ensure appropriate temperatures.
- Ensure appliances do not become a danger. Install devices that help to ensure safety, such as the automatic turn-off switch for your stove or oven. You may need to remove the control knobs on some, such as on the stove and microwave, or place signs saying broken, if its use becomes a danger.

Your **bathroom** now ranks high amongst areas in your home that require attention. There are many products available to transform your bathroom into one that is safe and sound. This list includes items such as:

- Install anti-scald devices in showers, tubs, and sinks (just like the device suggested for your kitchen sink.)
- If using a bathroom rug or mat, make sure it is anti-slip. Also, make sure to place an anti-slip mat or stickers inside the bathtub or shower.
- Use a safety plug to ensure the tub does not overfill.
- A commode chair for the toilet is recommended as it raises the height of the toilet seat and has armrests to assist in sitting and rising.
- I suggest using a bathtub or shower chair. Getting one that is a combo with a commode chair for the toilet is available and can save you money.
- Install grab/support rails anywhere extra support is needed, especially in the bathroom or stairwell.
- Use a transfer bench when necessary.
- A hand-held showerhead is a must.
- Consider converting your tub into a walk-in tub or shower.

It should not be at all surprising if, after reading these lists, you feel a bit overwhelmed. Realizing just how much needs to be done in order to prepare your home for your loved one and their safety may be a bit shocking. However, having all of this information provides you with a heads-up, which I believe, should be a great relief to you throughout your journey. This knowledge enables you to be proactive in making your home safe and ready for your loved one, throughout the various stages of this disease. Along with the list above, I have also created a comprehensive purchasing list with links to make this as easy as possible. Click the link or scan the QR code on the next page for the list and arm yourself with the tools you need for success. Link:https://bit.ly/3sGe9Ka.

To further provide an example of how important home safety can be, I will now share Jack's story.

Jack is a patient of mine. One night, Jack was doing laundry and left the detergent on top of the washing machine.

The next night, his grandma, a woman in her late seventies with dementia, got out of bed in the middle of the night. She was hungry and went to the kitchen to get something to eat. On her way, she apparently saw the detergent on top of the washing machine and thinking it was powdered milk, brought it into the kitchen and put it on the counter. She put several spoonfuls into a glass, mixed it with water, and drank the entire glass.

Needless to say, she became ill, and had to be taken to the emergency room. Her stomach needed to be pumped and she needed to be hooked up to several medications and fluids administered by IV drip. Luckily, she was otherwise in decent health and was able to survive. The doctor told Jack that she most likely would not have survived had her health not been what it was.

This is a real-life example of an accident caused by a simple case of leaving a poisonous substance within reach and this accident could have easily been avoided. Unfortunately, this book had not yet been written and Jack did not have the tools to set his house up for success.

This brings us to the topic of emergencies. Despite the best of preparations, accidents can happen, and you must make contingencies which will greatly diminish the risk of potential emergencies. Having a war chest filled with knowledge, will give you this step up - so prepare. Although we are talking about emergencies and accident prevention at this stage, anything can happen to create an emergency scenario, i.e.: heart attack, stroke, fall, etc. Keep a list of important emergency phone numbers, including emergency contacts, fire department, local police, poison control helplines, hospital, and 911. Although this might sound silly, people oftentimes freeze and are incapable of using their best judgment and are unable to think straight during a period of crisis. I have created an emergency binder for you. You can click this link: https://bit.ly/3MenDD9, if reading the e-book, or scan the QR code below if reading the print book to get your copy.

This a great tool to keep organized and have everything you need in one place in case of an emergency. This binder should be kept in an accessible place that is readily available, if needed, such as the fridge door.

Chapter 12
Managing Legalities and Financial Affairs

Whether it's planning for outside assistance, paying for expenses related to your loved one's care, insurance matters, social security, Medicare, or Medicaid, there is a lot to know. Managing legal matters and understanding available tax deductions, can provide you with additional assistance and hopefully enable you a better understanding of these potentially complex issues.

Hopefully, your loved one has already prepared a will, which would include naming a power of attorney, which will most probably be you, as the primary caregiver. This needs to be addressed while your loved one is still deemed to be legally competent. If you are not already a cosigner on their bank account or other financial institutions, this is the time to get it done. This also is the time to retain a financial advisor or accountant (if one is not already in place) who can help you understand your loved one's various assets and liabilities. Your advisor will be instrumental in aiding you in reviewing all financial plans already in place. An example, would be having a Roth IRA or other type of retirement plan. Your planner or accountant can determine if your loved one qualifies for tax-free exemptions, when withdrawing funds and will alert you of any required withdrawals.

Looking ahead is always important and it would be wise, at this time, to have your accountant or financial advisor provide you with a projection, which will allow you to better understand if the costs you will be facing will be of issue. As dementia is a progressive disease, at each stage, a person's needs will vary. Prescription drugs, personal care supplies, medical treatments (diagnosis, follow-up visits, etc.), adult day care services, in-home care services, safety-related expenditures, like home safety modification, and residential care services are among the more common costs associated with their care. Having a person you trust and can rely on to help advise you, will be of great assistance in preparing for any of these potential expenses.

Collect all relevant documents, organize them, and keep them in your binder under the legal documents section. Such documents would include: insurance policies, mortgage documents, bank account information, monthly bills, outstanding bills, medical and durable powers of attorney, rental income paperwork, stock and bond certificates, wills, and pension/retirement benefit summaries. A financial statement that indicates your loved one's assets and liabilities will be the first step in this process.

Insurance, such as Medicare, Medicaid (or state or country equivalent), disability insurance, group employee plans, long-term care insurance, and life insurance are avenues to explore. Government assistance and subsidies such as social security and veterans' benefits can also be important resources.

Your financial expert (financial advisor/accountant) will direct you to an attorney if there is additional assistance required to set up any of these legal documents.

If finances preclude you from having any of the above-mentioned professionals on board, you can seek assistance online, by visiting such sites as rocketlawyer.com, where you can draw up legal forms for free, such as designating a power of attorney. Although many professionals require a consultation fee, you may be able to find one that will offer a free consultation. You should use this opportunity to ask questions about state and country laws, to help you position yourself for the best possible outcome available.

The professionals you might seek include:

- Estate planning lawyer
- Elder-care lawyer
- Financial advisor/planner
- Accountant

If you are using a professional, the financial discussion should take place soon after the initial diagnosis.

Paying For Care

Once you have ascertained the care costs, it's time to come up with a game plan, to determine how you will be able to pay for it.

Your loved one, may be fortunate and have planned ahead by purchasing an at-home healthcare plan, long-term healthcare policy, and/or a long-term disability policy. These plans will be instrumental by providing you with daily benefits, which will aid in subsidizing at-home or facility-related care. If your loved one has one of these policies in place, be sure to read the fine print within the policy (or have one of your professionals review it), to verify whether the policy provides care in a facility, at home, or both. As part of this review, you should validate the daily or weekly allowance provided and confirm both the requirements and duration of the coverage.

Retirement plans, such as an individual retirement account (IRA) and/or annuities, can provide critical financial assistance, even if your loved one has not yet reached the required retirement age. If your loved one has an IRA, 401K, or other funds, you will need to find out if and how these funds can be pierced. If your loved one has a life insurance policy (universal/whole) that has built-up equity, this can be a source of income that can be drawn upon. You should also investigate the companies that offer to purchase existing policies. If you are living in your loved one's home and there is either no mortgage or there is built-up equity, you can look into refinancing the home and/or research reverse mortgages, to see if either would be beneficial.

Another avenue to explore, is the type of insurance your loved one qualifies for, i.e.: Medicare or Medicaid (check your country/state-specific titles for government-provided insurance). If you live in the United States, at age 65, you are eligible to receive Medicare. For many people, this is the main source of healthcare coverage.

If your loved one has assets, you should share this with your financial advisor/accountant/attorney, so that they can help you determine whether or not you are legally able to void these assets, in order to qualify for government assistance. Your financial advisor/accountant/attorney can determine whether you need to take steps that will ensure your loved one will qualify and not be denied benefits based upon these assets. Reminder, this must be done with ample forethought, as there is a timed look-back period (5 years), which is set in place to ensure that people are truly eligible for government assistance and not just ridding themselves of assets, in order to qualify.

There may be personal resources belonging to your loved one that can serve as a source of income and therefore, be used to pay for care. Examples could be personal property used as rentals and/or investments.

Community support services may be available and are provided by non-profit organizations. These services can be free or offered at a low cost and can provide respite care, transportation, home-delivered meals, support groups, etc.

Insurance - a More Detailed Look

The United States government offers various programs such as Medicare, Medicaid (AKA Medi-Cal in California - check your country/state-specific equivalent), Medicare Advantage, and Medigap Insurance.

Medicare is a federal health insurance program for people age 65 and older, or for people who are younger than 65 and are receiving Social Security disability benefits for at least 24 months.

Medicare Advantage allows you to choose Medicare Health Maintenance Organization (HMO), Point of Service (POS), and Preferred Provider Organization (PPO), effectively letting you control managed care costs.

Medigap insurance supplements your Medicare coverage - fills the "gaps" in Original Medicare Plan coverage.

Medicaid is funded by both the federal and state governments and is administered by each state, which qualifies individuals with low income and minimal assets, for additional medical assistance, as well as long-term care.

Supplemental Security Income is another benefit that is available. To qualify, one must have minimal income and resources and be age 65 or older, or have a disability, such as dementia, wherein the age limit is not a restriction.

If a **long-term care insurance policy** is already in place when diagnosed, benefits covered by this policy will be enforceable.

Approximately 60-70 percent of your loved one's gross income can be provided by a **disability insurance policy**. This type of insurance is for a worker who is disabled because of an illness or injury and can no longer continue to work. Just as with long-term insurance, this type of insurance must already be in place before dementia is diagnosed. The policy should be checked, to review what is covered and for how long, as most disability policies convert to social security at age 65.

If your loved one has **life insurance,** check to see if their policy offers an accelerated death benefit. If you have a universal/whole life policy and have built-up equity, you may be able to borrow against it, without incurring penalties or having to pay back the withdrawn portion of your built-up equity. However, be sure, as always, to check the fine print in your policy or make it easy on yourself - call your agent or have your professional advisor review the policy.

Medicare

Medicare is a US federal health insurance program for people who are 65 or older or younger and have a qualifying disability or health condition.

Medicare consists of three parts:

Medicare Part A (Hospital Insurance) covers inpatient hospital stays, care in a skilled nursing facility, hospice care, and some home health care.

Medicare Part B (Medical Insurance) covers certain services received from healthcare providers, doctors, outpatient care, medical supplies, and preventive services.

Medicare Part D (Prescription Drug Coverage) helps to cover the cost of prescription drugs (including many recommended injections and vaccines).

Medicare Part C (Medicare Managed Care) are health plan options offered by private companies approved by Medicare. They provide both Part A and Part B coverage and may include additional benefits such as vision, hearing, dental, and wellness programs, which include point of service plans (POS), preferred provider organizations (PPO), and Medicare Health Maintenance Organizations (HMO).

If you have Medicare, it is suggested that you acquire supplemental insurance (**Medigap**), which is an additional insurance policy that covers any deductibles and copayments not already paid by Medicare. Note, that supplemental insurance only becomes applicable when Medicare has already approved the claim.

Medicaid

As previously mentioned, Medicaid is available for people who have both minimal income and assets. Medicaid pays for all medical care, including long-term care. It's funded by both the federal and state governments. Medicaid covers all or some portion of nursing home costs for end-of-life patients, though there's a caveat here because not all nursing homes accept Medicaid. To apply for Medicaid, you have to contact the Department of Welfare or the Department of Health. They will seek information that determines your loved one's financial need and whether or not they qualify.

Steve, one of my patients, told me about his aunt, whose niece was her caregiver. They were searching for any assistance available to them and found that they were able to qualify for financial assistance for home care through Medi-Cal. Medi-Cal is California's version of Medicaid. Although Medi-Cal is specific to California, each state has its own similar program. If your loved one qualifies for Medi-Cal, then they automatically would be eligible to apply for at-home care. In this case, Medi-Cal would send a qualified professional to the home to determine the level of care required and based upon that, will determine the hours deemed necessary and the allotted dollar amount per hour. Steve told me that his aunt qualified for 6 hours a day and the payment was based on the prevailing caregiver rate. They were provided bi-monthly time sheets that had to be filled out and signed, and thereafter, a check was dispersed. He told me that this money was to pay for the provider of care and that the provider could be either an outside person or, in this case, his aunt's niece, the caregiver. Steve said that this money was instrumental in allowing his aunt to remain living in her home, by providing her niece with supplemental income, so that she could afford to quit her job and make caregiving her full-time commitment.

Tax Deductions

Tax deductions vary from state to state and country to country and it's best to check with your accountant to determine all benefits you may be eligible for, as the primary caregiver.

If your loved one has sufficient income and assets, they are entitled to include any of the medical and dementia-related expenses as deductions on their tax returns. If you, the caregiver, are being paid to be the caregiver for your loved one, the expenses that you pay for, might be deductible as well. As always, consult with your accountant or professional for the best way to proceed. There are cases where you can assume guardianship, which may also help to reduce the amount of taxes owed to Uncle Sam; however, this is a complicated issue and you will need to seek professional advice to determine if this would apply to your situation.

At the risk of sounding redundant, I want to urge you to discuss any and all questions related to these matters with an expert - financial advisor, accountant, or attorney.

Legal Matters

Hopefully, by now, your loved one has their will and all other long-term, end-of-life decisions in place. Your legal planning should include preparation for short and long-term care, as well as, other healthcare needs, including but not limited to naming an executor and having a power of attorney in place. In a perfect world, this has been done prior to your loved one having any sign of dementia, so that family members and others are unable to challenge the competence and capability of your loved one when making such decisions. Having these documents in your possession also confirms that your loved one was involved when making all of these related decisions.

These items include:

- Estate planning documents such as wills, trusts, and powers of attorney
- Real estate deeds
- List of assets, as well as their owners and beneficiaries for items, including: safe deposit boxes, vehicles, bank accounts, real estate, etc.
- Copies of income tax returns
- Long-term care insurance policies and other similar policies, including home health care
- Life insurance policies

By having all of these documents prior to the onset of their diagnosis, as stated above, the risk of having any of the decisions challenged, will be greatly minimized.

Legal Documents

The aforementioned legal documents described in the previous section—power of attorney, living will, power of attorney for health care, and living trust—are amongst the documents that will ensure your loved one's wishes are followed, even when the disease has progressed, and they are no longer able to make such decisions. Many of these documents will differ from state to state, country to country.

Power of Attorney

A power of attorney is a document you should be sure to create just as the term indicates, it allows for the maker to designate a person to make any and all decisions in the event the creator is unable to do so (as in the case of a person with dementia). The person named as power of attorney, should be aware of their designation and should be familiar and knowledgeable with regard to assets, liabilities, and care directives, such as the living will, which includes a DNR (do not resuscitate order), if applicable, and any trusts. This designation is air-tight and, if necessary, will hold up in a court of law. It would be prudent to have a backup person in place, in the event the designated power of attorney, you, are no longer able to provide such service.

Power of Attorney for Health Care - Advanced Directive

This document serves as does the power of attorney, we just reviewed; however, it is a limited, specific power that relates only to healthcare issues and is commonly known as an advanced directive. If your loved one is in a hospital or healthcare facility, you, the caregiver, will most likely be asked to provide this document, as it would allow you to make all health and life-altering decisions regarding care provided to your loved one. This would include decisions such as resuscitation (if a do-not-resuscitate - DNR is not already in place), as well as any potential surgeries, tube feeding, etc.

Living Will

A living will is another type of advance directive that ensures the creator's wishes are honored with regard to medical decisions. This document further guarantees that your loved one's desires are respected and should be retained along with their power of attorney and be included with all their other legal documents and placed in the legal section of your binder.

Standard Will

A standard will, names the executor, who will be responsible for ensuring that all of your loved one's wishes are honored with respect to all of the terms of the will. Within this document, a beneficiary or beneficiaries will be named, and it will be their responsibility to ensure that all assets are distributed in the designated fashion your loved one has chosen. This includes any money or other financial assets, as well as real estate and personal belongings and can be so descriptive as to include, even their most favorite chachkas, such as a silver-handled hair brush, figurine, etc.

Living Trust

A living trust is a form of estate planning that allows you to control your assets (your money and property) while you are still alive and indicates the people and/or organizations designated to be beneficiaries upon your death. There are many reasons to create a living trust. Discuss the pros and cons of creating such a document with an attorney who specializes in wills, estates, and trusts. Tax-related advantages often dictate whether or not you decide to create a living trust.

Guardianship/Conservatorship

If a person with dementia is deemed unable to make their own care decisions and they do not have the necessary aforementioned documents in place, a guardian or conservator will be appointed by the court to make the decisions regarding their assets and care.

I included this important chapter to ensure you are provided with the information necessary when navigating your loved one's financial affairs, legalities, insurance, and tax-related matters. This is a crucial component and provides an essential tool for you, the caregiver. Understanding such complexities paves the way, allowing you to shift your focus on what really matters - caregiving for your loved one.

Although we have already reviewed many treatments and medications available, in the next two chapters, I will share lifestyle modifications for you and your loved one to ensure you both can maintain a healthy life and potentially slow your loved one's progression of dementia. I will also introduce holistic approaches, as well as diets and supplements, which will be great additions to your care regimen.

Chapter 13
Lifestyle Modifications

There are varying views as to whether or not dementia is hereditary, as some forms of dementia, i.e., Alzheimer's, are believed to be such. Therefore, if one of your close family members has suffered from dementia, it may be of great concern to you, with regard to your own health. The thought of having dementia is scary and creates great fear, especially if as the caregiver, you have witnessed this firsthand.

Although dementia is a progressive disease and currently cannot be reversed, it doesn't necessarily have to be as bleak as we have been led to believe. You can do more than sit around and pray for some miracle medical cure to be discovered. You should not be discouraged from implementing research-based strategies, which can possibly slow down the process of mental and physical deterioration. With all the research and continued knowledge regarding this disease, hopefully, in the months and years to come, continued strides will be made and an eventual cure will be discovered, in our lifetime. To allay the concerns and fears you may be experiencing regarding this disease, I am sharing strategies that can both slow down the aggressive progression for your loved one, as well as, be implemented by you, to reduce your risk of developing this disease.

How, you ask?

Dementia is a very complex disease with more than one risk factor. Some of these factors are totally outside of your or your loved one's control, such as genetics and age. Lifestyle habits such as smoking, drinking, diet, exercise, and mental well-being are in your control and can be a great place to start.

Researchers believe that there are seven factors that can reduce the risk of developing dementia and help your loved one delay the onset of its more severe symptoms. These seven factors are:

- Physical exercise
- Social interaction
- Healthy diet
- Mental stimulation
- Maintaining quality sleep
- Managing stress
- Vascular health

Physical Exercise

According to the Alzheimer's Research and Prevention Foundation, consistent physical exercise is known to reduce one's risk of developing dementia, by as much as 50%. Regular exercise is known to slow down the deterioration of the disease. Exercise stimulates the brain and can help in maintaining old connections, as well as allowing for new connections to be made, which can delay the progression of dementia. The key is that there must be consistency. This does not mean you must exercise daily; however, consider exercising several times each week. Cardio and strength training should be included in your mix of exercises.

Swimming is great and is the equivalent of moderately intense exercise. Many people are unable to take a brisk walk and may suffer from joint pain, including arthritis. Others may be immobile, but regardless of their situation, there is always a form of exercise available. For these people, swimming, chair yoga, or a form of water aerobics may be perfect alternatives, as it is a non-weight-bearing exercise. You should commit to exercising with your loved one and make it a scheduled activity. This will help keep both you and your loved one physically active.

The benefits of physical exercise are vast, it helps to maintain and build muscle (avoiding atrophy), improve strength, balance, and coordination, and maintain brain health and cognitive function. As stated by the Mayo Clinic, "Exercise in any form acts as a stress reliever. Being active can boost your feel-good endorphins and distract you from daily worries."

So pick your poison, swimming, walking, yoga, tai chi, etc. The choice is yours, but don't delay - start today!

Social Interaction

Human beings are wired to be social creatures. Isolation can do a number on mental health. Remaining socially engaged and having interactions with others, can help slow down the progression of the disease.

If your loved one is mobile, you can take them to a local shelter or soup kitchen where you can team together and perform simple tasks. This will not only be an activity that benefits them, but also can provide a feeling of being needed, by those less fortunate. Tailor the social activity to align with interests they have enjoyed in the past. As an example, if they like to read, consider joining a book club. Any social gathering where they have the opportunity to be with like-minded people is sure to offer social interaction and companionship and elevate their mood.

Many assisted living facilities and community centers, such as senior centers, have programs available. Availing yourself of these opportunities, will give your loved one a chance to be with people their age and will provide a means for them to share experiences and engage in conversation. Since time is often limited, you can get creative and combine social and physical activities, by finding an appropriate group class for things such as: aerobics, yoga, and tai chi. There are endless possibilities when it comes to social activities. To make it more enjoyable, find one that both you and your loved one enjoy.

A Healthy Diet

Insulin resistance and inflammatory conditions damage and debilitate communication between the neurons. This is why Alzheimer's and dementia are known as the diabetes of the mind. New research has uncovered a direct correlation between metabolic disorders (i.e., diabetes) and the brain's signal-processing systems. With this revelation, it has become evident that healthy eating habits can reduce inflammation, thereby preserving metabolic function, which can potentially prevent the occurrence of the disease or delay its progression.

There are various diets that have been proven to be effective in combating dementia and can prevent or slow its symptoms. Although there are many, there is one diet I highly recommend. This diet is rich in non-starchy vegetables, olive oil, beans, fish, fruit, poultry, whole grains, nuts, berries, and leafy greens. This diet is the MIND diet (Mediterranean-DASH Intervention for Neurodegenerative Decay). The MIND diet is known to reduce the decline in brain health, thus reducing the risk of dementia and/or slowing down dementia-associated mental deterioration. The MIND diet prohibits the consumption of butter, margarine, pastries, sweets, fried food, red meat, and cheese, as these foods contain saturated fats, trans fats, and sugar, all of which contribute to diseases, including dementia.

Whether or not you are willing to follow the MIND diet, please be sure, at a minimum, to provide you and your loved one with a balanced diet that contains the aforementioned recommended foods. It is also very important to eliminate or limit foods that are high in saturated fat, simple carbohydrates, and foods that contain refined sugar, and those that are high in sodium.

Limiting foods like pasta, white rice, white flour, cane sugar, etc., is important, as they have a negative impact on blood sugar and can lead to inflammation of both your body and brain.

Another benefit of a healthy diet relates to weight. Research has determined that people who are clinically obese in midlife are three times more likely to develop dementia, later on in life.

Eat food rich in Omega-3 fats. Omega-3 fats contain DHA (Docosahexaenoic Acid), which is known to prevent and/or slow down dementia. Other benefits of Omega-3 fats are that it helps to reduce the risk of heart disease, can improve ADHD, fights inflammation, supports muscle development and its recovery, and is even known to reduce the risk of many forms of cancer.

Foods that are high in Omega-3 fats include: cold-water fish, such as trout, sardines, salmon, and tuna. In lieu of fish, you can add a fish oil supplement, which can be found in varying forms, including pills. Some, will have an aftertaste, so look for the "burpless" options. As always, when adding any new over-the-counter medication, vitamin, or supplement, check with your doctor or pharmacist to ensure that there will be no negative interactions with any medications currently taken.

If your loved one is prone to drinking, now would be the time for them to stop. Alcohol consumption drastically accelerates brain aging and also increases the risk of developing dementia.

Mental Stimulation

Whether you're looking to delay the progression of dementia in your loved one or prevent it altogether for yourself or someone close to you, it's important to understand that when it comes to the brain, it's a case of "use it or lose it." It is important to stimulate the brain by challenging your mind in whatever capacity is possible, no matter what age you are. Older adults, who keep their minds stimulated, preserve cognitive functioning and exhibit a significant delay in brain aging, which is referenced in the NIH ACTIVE study.

If possible, join your loved one in learning something new. This can include such things as playing a musical instrument, learning a new language, painting, coloring, puzzles, sewing, knitting, or even cooking (with constant supervision, of course). These activities will not only slow down the progression of dementia by helping to keep the brain mentally active for as long as possible, but will also aid in preserving independence.

Maintaining Quality Sleep

As quoted by Francesca Annis, "The minute anyone's getting anxious, I say, you must eat and you must sleep. They're the two vital elements for a healthy life."

Poor sleeping patterns are associated with the development of dementia. In addition, it is a contributing factor in the increased speed of progression in patients who have already started showing symptoms. When a person has consistently good quality sleep, their body flushes out toxins in their brain and reduces the levels of beta-amyloid, which is a sticky protein that can disrupt deep sleep. Deep sleep is essential for memory formation.

Getting quality sleep is paramount for your loved one, as it slows down the progression of the disease and regulates their energy levels. To assist them with their sleep, establish a regular schedule so that their internal clock (natural circadian rhythm) kicks in.

In order to accomplish this, set the mood by dimming the lights and pulling the blinds. In the bedroom, there should be no visual distractions, such as TVs, phones, and screens. The bedroom should be a special place reserved for sleeping.

Assist your loved one with a bedtime ritual. A nice hot bath, minor stretching, listening to calming music, or reading a few pages of their favorite book will send a powerful signal to their mind that it's time for some deep sleep.

If all else fails, consult with your doctor to determine if the addition of a sleep aid would be beneficial.

If your loved one tends to snore or you notice a disruption in their breathing while they sleep, I suggest you have them screened for sleep apnea. Sleep apnea is another culprit that can disrupt deep sleep - besides being potentially dangerous. When treated, the quality of sleep will improve.

Managing Stress

You, as the caregiver, have a huge amount on your plate. Worrying about your loved one (and yourself) and the future can cause added anxiety and stress. You and or your loved one can also be dealing with mental health issues, including depression and the jarring realization that life is changing, and in the case of your loved one, their abilities are gradually or rapidly declining. When such mental stress strains the brain, it can shrink key memory areas and stop nerve cell growth, both of which can increase the speed of deterioration.

Although you both may be taking specific medications from your doctor to treat agitation, anxiety, and depression; without stress management, you may not succeed, as medication alone may not be the sole fix for these issues. A visit to a therapist might be a more meaningful recommendation to you, the caregiver, as it would provide a person to whom you can vent and confide your fears and concerns. If your loved one is in the earlier throws of this disease, having them visit with a therapist, could also be beneficial.

Breathing exercises have been shown to improve stress relief. There are many other forms of release that can help to reduce stress, as well. To name a few: meditation, mindfulness exercises, progressive muscular relaxation, yoga, music therapy, art therapy, and talk therapy. Laughter is known to be a great stress reliever - laugh hard and laugh often. These suggestions are beneficial to both you and your loved one.

If you and or your loved one are religious, consider creating spiritual and religious activities and/or invite someone from your house of worship to visit. This could go a long way in achieving inner peace by reigniting your faith in a higher power and your religion.

Vascular Health

Cardiovascular risk factors such as high cholesterol, hypertension, obesity, and atherosclerosis increase the risk of dementia, as well as cause rapid neurodegeneration.

Research-based evidence suggests that everything good for the heart is also good for the brain. When we maintain our and our loved one's cardiovascular health, we are paving the way to protect the brain and slow down neurodegeneration. By implementing the above lifestyle suggestions (i.e.: healthy diet, exercise, stress reduction, etc.), blood pressure and cholesterol levels should result in a marked improvement.

Although we have already addressed the negatives of drinking, smoking is yet another vice, that is just as, or even more harmful. If possible, remove all cigarettes and smoking devices. If quitting cold turkey is not a possibility, get creative. Replacing actual cigarettes with a fake substitute can satisfy the hand-to-mouth sensation and just might do the trick. If additional intervention is necessary, I suggest that you consult with your doctor or pharmacist, as there are many available treatments. Another option, would be to seek the assistance of a hypnotherapist. Quitting smoking will improve blood circulation and reduce the level of toxins and harmful chemicals in the bloodstream. It not only will help to slow down the progression of dementia, but will also help in improving vascular health.

Vascular health can also be improved with a healthy diet, which includes foods that are rich in fiber, fish, nuts, dark chocolate, and tea. Omitting or limiting salt, sugar, alcohol, and saturated fats, which are not healthy, can go a long way in improving vascular health. The Dietary Approach to Stop Hypertension (DASH) is one such diet that lowers blood pressure (hypertension) and is widely recognized in the medical field. This diet is rich in calcium, magnesium, potassium, and protein. Note that the MIND diet discussed previously, is a hybrid of the DASH and Mediterranean diets.

In this chapter, we reviewed lifestyle changes that you and your loved one can implement. We looked at strategies that can help improve both your and your loved one's health by increasing physical and social activities. We addressed the importance of quality sleep along with a quality diet. I provided tips for you to employ, in order to engage your loved one in activities to keep their mind active and stimulated, as well as tips to reduce stress. Armed with this knowledge, you should have a better understanding of how vascular health relates to brain health, and why it is so important.

There are also alternative treatments available, which include various types of therapies, which I address in the following chapter.

Chapter 14
Holistic and Alternative Care

What is Holistic Care?

Holistic healthcare includes alternative medicine, Eastern-inspired treatments, and naturopathy, a system of treatment that avoids drugs and surgery and emphasizes the use of natural agents. A more accurate description of holistic care is that it cares for the whole person, rather than just focusing on the disease's symptoms. This includes spiritual, mental, physical, and social needs. The basis behind these treatments, is that any one aspect can affect overall health, and if any of these aspects are affected, it can impact other areas as well.

Dementia oftentimes results in feelings of frustration, depression, confusion, anger, and anxiousness. Holistic and other forms of alternative care, not only cater to medical needs, but also provide positive reinforcements to support emotional needs. Holistic and other forms of alternative care, approach dementia as a whole-body experience, specifically centering around four things—language, activity, nutrition, and environment.

Although we have previously addressed how nutrition, environment, and language are integral for the mental peace of your loved one, we will now explore how activities and therapies combined can additionally enhance your loved one's care plan. This will further ensure that your loved one is able to live a more meaningful and fulfilling life; while discouraging negative feelings derived from boredom, loneliness, and depression.

Different Forms of Holistic Care

The most effective and prominent holistic care methods include:

- Massage Therapy
- Acupuncture
- Yoga
- Neurofeedback Therapy
- Cognitive Behavioral Therapy
- Cannabis Therapy
- Pet Therapy
- Music Therapy
- Art Therapy
- Gardening Therapy
- Aromatherapy
- Exercising

Why do I suggest incorporating some or all of these forms of therapies?

I believe that by caring for your loved one's well-being as a whole, you will be better able to help restore balance in all aspects of their health. Holistic care has far fewer potential side effects compared to Western medicine. Although it is important that your loved one receives the necessary medication and does so as prescribed by your doctor, it is quite possible that holistic and alternative non-prescription medications can alleviate some symptoms without associated side effects.

Although often overlooked, these therapies have tremendous value. You would be surprised how various forms of massage therapy and acupuncture may aid with the chronic pain associated with dementia, especially vascular dementia. Art and music therapy can offer a dual service, not only by alleviating stress and disassociation but also keeping their mind active, providing enjoyment, and elevating self-esteem. This is especially true if these are areas of interest and or passions they have enjoyed throughout their life.

Massage Therapy

Vascular dementia mimics symptoms of a stroke, which can manifest as causing the fingers to curl and the hand to become clenched. Physiotherapy and massage therapy can help these extremities return to normal function.

Whether or not your loved one exhibits these symptoms, massage therapy can also relieve symptoms associated with agitation, anxiety, and depression, while simultaneously providing pain relief. The core element at the center of massage therapy is its human connection. Interaction with your loved one through the powerful, meditative, and physical action of massage, not only relieves pain but also provides the soothing connection of touch. Touch can be an important tool in helping to eliminate feelings of isolation.

Massage therapy has also been associated with a variety of other benefits, including, but not limited to:

- Assisting in both helping one fall asleep as well as enjoy a better nights sleep
- Regulating blood pressure and heart rate
- Eliminating/reducing physical discomfort (muscle pain and tightness)
- Reducing overall stress levels
- Strengthening the immune system
- Improving circulation
- Promoting relaxation, thereby causing levels of stress hormones to decrease
- Improving joint mobility and mobility-related conditions, such as bed sores
- Increasing flexibility
- Improving the recovery rate of soft tissue injuries

Specific massages can address other issues. For example, an abdominal massage can relieve constipation.

There are many types of massage therapies.

- **Swedish massage** is a full-body massage that calms the nervous system
- **Deep tissue massage** is meant to relieve pain in muscles and tendons
- **Trigger point massage** works on knots in the neck and chronic back pain, as well as pain in the legs

and arms

- **Myofascial release** centers on the connective tissue under the skin and is meant to relieve tension and tightness throughout the body
- **Lymphatic massage** stimulates the lymphatic system and drastically reduces inflammation, such as in the case of arthritis

Acupuncture

Acupuncture is part of traditional Chinese medicine (TCM), in which a practitioner uses fine needles to stimulate different anatomic areas, known as acupuncture points, under the skin surface. This is used to improve the flow of Qi (pronounced Chee), thereby improving one's health. Qi is the energy flow throughout the body that's responsible for maintaining overall health.

Aside from dementia, other symptoms and disorders that acupuncture treatments include: stroke rehabilitation, osteoarthritis, lower back pain, carpal tunnel syndrome, myofascial pain, and fibromyalgia.

Research has shown that acupuncture plays a role in improving circulation to the brain. It improves both brain function and oxygen flow while reducing stress hormones such as cortisol and increases dopamine, acetylcholine (a neurotransmitter specific to memory), and serotonin.

Beta-amyloid plaques, a sticky protein known to be responsible for cognitive decline, as it accumulates in the brain, causes a reduction of blood flow. This increased toxin build-up causes oxidative stress, which inflames the brain, all of which compounds the issues associated with dementia.

These beta-amyloids are removed through acupuncture, cleaning the brain and allowing it to do its job more effectively. Acupuncture stimulates the central nervous system by releasing chemicals in the brain, spinal cord, and muscles, which in turn stimulates the body's natural healing ability and promotes both emotional and physical well-being.

Yoga

You may already know how yoga's meditative properties can help calm the mind, while its physical aspect can improve strength and build flexibility. But, did you also know that yoga can be beneficial in both assisting, as well as delaying symptoms of dementia? In a single-blind controlled study of seniors, researchers discovered that those who practiced yoga showed marked improvement both in immediate and delayed memory recall. In addition, yoga has been shown to increase blood circulation, respiration, and range of motion and can improve balance. All of these benefits can help to prevent falls and prolong mobility. By practicing yoga, one becomes more aware of their body, space, and movement.

Yoga also can indirectly increase the ability to deal with pain. The spiritual aspect of yoga is meant to improve one's sense of well-being, as it can be beneficial in regulating emotions and can elevate one's mood. Interestingly, yoga is also known to increase the presence of telomerase, which is the enzyme that is responsible for slowing down cell aging. Besides these dementia-related benefits, yoga is also known to improve sleep, improve breathing, boost heart health, enhance body flexibility, build muscle, and reduce mental strain, often caused by depression, stress, and anxiety.

With all of these benefits, it is no wonder that Yoga has become extremely popular. The easy learning curve makes it accessible for anyone, regardless of age and mobility.

Neurofeedback Therapy

EEG Biofeedback Therapy, also known as Neurofeedback Therapy, is a non-drug therapy that facilitates patients to regulate their brain activity and self-generate healthier brainwave patterns to improve memory, emotional recognition, and, most importantly, cognitive function.

Alpha waves are known to bring about meditativeness, peacefulness, readiness, and deep relaxation, whereas beta waves are associated with focus, attention, tension, excitement, and alertness.

In this form of therapy, electrodes connected to your brain (placed over your head non-invasively) provide immediate feedback on brainwave activity. When you manifest alpha or beta waves, the screen brightens, letting you know that you're succeeding. It's almost like a game where your main focus is to keep the screen shining bright with the power of your mind.

When one suffers from dementia, the neurons and neural pathways are damaged. Although it is not possible for the brain damage to be reversed through neurofeedback therapy, the symptoms can be better managed.

As far as holistic therapies go, neurofeedback therapy is a great option, in that it's non-invasive, there is no reliance on drugs, it allows the patient to self-regulate their brain activity by teaching how to produce alpha and beta waves, and it improves mood, emotional stability, cognitive functioning, concentration, impulse control, memory, and organizational skills. Moreover, as with other holistic therapies, it can be used as a stand-alone therapy or in combination with other treatments.

Cognitive Behavioral Therapy (CBT)

A technique primarily used for helping people with dementia manage mental health issues such as anxiety, depression, poor concentration, and sleeplessness. During this therapy, the patient will be asked questions to elicit how they think in a given situation and how that situation affects them. Gradually, through these therapy sessions, the goal is to divert any negative mindset that presents itself, into a healthy and more positive emotional response - commonly known as behavioral modification.

As dementia is a neurological condition and not a mental illness, cognitive behavioral therapy cannot treat the disease or reverse it. However, it can be helpful to treat the mental health symptoms associated with the disease.

CBT has many benefits in helping dementia patients

- Treating anxiety and depression can be helpful in boosting self-esteem and creating a sense of independence
- Assisting with long-term memory recall and facilitating interactions with friends and family
- Improving the immune system
- Promoting a better sense of self-awareness, as well as coping skills

- Tackling the psychological morbidity associated with dementia

CBT can be an asset when preparing your loved one to face the challenges that lie ahead and, hopefully, will assist you in coming to an acceptable perspective.

Cannabis Therapy

Given the limited, currently available therapeutic options, their side-effect profiles, and inconsistent evidence base, there is a need for alternative therapies, in our growing population of dementia patients. Medical cannabis has been researched, and studies indicate that it is a potential alternative treatment for dementia. Cannabis (also known as marijuana) is a medicinal plant comprised of both cannabinoids and terpenes, all of which have therapeutic benefits.

Limited evidence from one systematic review and one uncontrolled before-and-after study suggests that medical cannabis may be effective for treating agitation, disinhibition, irritability, aberrant motor behavior, and nocturnal behavioral disorders, as well as aberrant vocalization and resting care, which are neuropsychiatric symptoms associated with dementia.

Due to cannabis's medical-legal classification in many states, there are more and more doctors and pharmacists who are well-versed in cannabis medicine. They can assist in helping treat your loved one's symptoms with cannabis. They can also determine if there are any drug interactions that you would need to be aware of and assist you in finding the correct product, form, and dose.

Medical marijuana is now legal in many states and countries (check your state and or country laws) and is currently prescribed by more and more doctors to reduce inflammation, treat anxiety disorders, prevent drug relapses, lower blood pressure, treat gastrointestinal disorders, prevent seizures, fight cancer, treat epilepsy, sclerosis, deal with chronic pain, provide symptom relief in palliative care, and so much more.

Compared to opioids and other prescribed drugs, marijuana has more benefits and fewer side effects and risks. When given for pain relief, it does not heavily sedate and debilitate the recipient as much as its counterparts (opioids) do. Opioids pose many risks in dementia patients and cannabis offers an alternative solution. To date, a fatal overdose of cannabis has never been documented and is considered impossible.

Studies have shown that many patients prefer to treat psychological morbidity with medical marijuana instead of resorting to drugs like lorazepam, clonazepam, sertraline, trazodone, and bupropion.

Cannabis is a plant medicine and comes in a variety of strains and types (edibles, tinctures, vape pens, etc.). With so many variants of cannabis therapy available, there is something for everyone. Patients can avail the benefits of the drug without having to get high, as CBD, one of the main cannabinoids, is a non-psychoactive compound that is responsible for many of these benefits. CBD does not get a person "high." Rather, it's THC, another cannabinoid, which is responsible for this psychoactive component.

Cannabis can not only help to reduce stress, anxiety, and insomnia for your loved one, but it can do the same for you, the caregiver.

One thing to caution, is that many edible forms of cannabis come in attractive packaging and can also come in the form of candy, cookies, or cake; it is therefore extremely important that you lock up these edible forms of cannabis, to prevent accidental ingestion. I recommend avoiding edibles as the effect can be delayed and more intense and can contain sugar and other additives, for oral preparations, tinctures are my preferred choice as it is easier to control the dosage and they tend to contain less sugar and additives.

Pet Therapy

In recent years, animal-assisted therapy has been getting great press and has been rightfully credited, especially for its success with dementia patients. Dr. William Thompson, has been credited for his theory of integrating pets, plants, and children into elder-care facilities for dementia patients. His goal was to improve the patient's mood and help them battle helplessness, loneliness, and boredom.

Does this theory hold weight? Yes, it does. Pet therapy is proven to be very beneficial for dementia patients. For starters, it improves mood and provides an opportunity for social interaction. Taking care of an animal can provide a sense of purpose, as well as, reduce anxiety and can increase physical activity; all, while elevating your loved one's sense of need and mood. In a 2008 study, psychologists observed that pet therapy had a very calming effect on nursing home residents. Moreover, studies have shown that pet therapy can lower blood pressure, while offering an element of companionship.

Music Therapy

Music is universal and can be enjoyed in a multitude of languages and is the world's greatest connector. Oliver Sacks, best-selling author and professor of neurology, at N.Y.U. School Of Medicine, said it best, when he said: "Music can lift us out of depression or move us to tears – it is a remedy, a tonic, orange juice for the ear. But for many of my neurological patients, music is even more – it can provide access, even when no medication can, to movement, to speech, to life. For them, music is not a luxury, but a necessity."

Music accesses different parts of the brain and can be a tool of communication for engaging with a loved one with dementia. Even if your loved one is not capable of responding verbally, music can transcend this barrier of diminished speech. Calming music can evoke a soothing emotional reaction. Familiar music or special songs from childhood or earlier years, can tap into powerful emotions and memories. Music can also assist in facilitating physical exercise in the form of dance, aerobics, or just simple movements. Who doesn't love a sing-a-long? Hopefully, no one you know! Seriously, joining your loved one in a simple, well-known song or doing the same when you have a guest(s) visiting can drastically reduce social isolation and is sure to bring a smile to your loved one's face.

Art Therapy

Art therapy can stimulate the mind, while also being a fun and relaxing way for your loved one to express creativity. Whether it's paint, crayons, or any other type of medium, participants in art therapy have been known to show cognitive and behavioral improvement. Art therapy is known to trigger dormant memories that can allow your loved one to enjoy the memories of yesteryear, that for so long have been forgotten. Given the subjective nature of art and the fact that art is not a case where one size fits all, it's all about choosing whatever form of art resonates with your loved one. I encourage you to participate as art therapy is a great way to relieve stress, and as a caregiver, I'm sure you have some spare stress to color away.

Gardening / Horticulture Therapy

Gardening or horticulture therapy is normally performed in a garden or yard. It is a holistic method that has shown great benefit to people dealing with symptoms of dementia. If you can't bring your loved one to the garden, you can bring the garden to them!

Interacting with nature has very therapeutic effects on people, even if they're simply viewing trees or visiting gardens. There's a connecting sense of healing, which is felt when growing things. In essence, gardening therapy works by promoting confidence, improving communication skills, strengthening memory and cognition, boosting the immune system, and thereby, enhancing your loved one's mood.

This type of therapy, which I call "group therapy," is a favorite of mine because the whole family can share and participate. If your loved one is still at a stage where they have some recognition, they can watch their flowers and plants grow, and as they do, your loved one will most assuredly take pleasure and enjoy watching as their colors change and they become more beautiful. This therapy is well-recognized by elder-care facilities. Many have communal gardens for this exact purpose.

Horticulture therapy, aka gardening, is considered to be a meditative/holistic activity. It promotes a sense of calmness, stimulates the senses, and provides a connection to Mother Nature. This therapy also aids in the reduction of blood pressure, stress, anxiety, anger, sadness, and fear. And, simply by the "nature" of this activity, your loved one and you will be spending time in the open air, which alone would be enough to brighten both of your days!

Aromatherapy

Aromatherapy uses scented essential oils from herbs, flowers, and plants to improve one's mental and physical health. It works by stimulating our olfactory receptors. For instance, bergamot, lemon balm, and lavender are useful to dementia patients as they increase sleep duration, reduce agitation, and create a sense of calm. Eucalyptus oil can be used to treat the symptoms of the common cold. These oils can be used to massage, can be added to baths, or sprinkled on pillows.

Although I don't want to get too technical, many of the benefits of aromatherapy come from terpenes. Yes, these are the same terpenes in cannabis. Terpenes are naturally occurring chemical compounds that can be found in plants and are responsible for the aromas, flavors, and even the colors associated with various types of vegetation.

Aromatherapy also has many health benefits, such as: improved sleep, stress reduction, pain management, etc., and can also be of great enjoyment for both you and your loved one.

Exercising

I know, I have previously discussed the importance of exercise. It is so beneficial to you and your loved one, which is why I felt it worthy of another mention. Any form of physical exercise can improve cardiovascular fitness and endurance, build strength, help to maintain motor skills, and prevent atrophy. Physical exercise can also serve to reduce the rate of cognitive decline. Physical exertion can elevate mood, regulate sleep, and possibly may even reduce the likelihood of constipation. Exercise can be done from a bed or chair, if your loved one is not mobile.

Although we know that there is no way to reverse or eliminate the decline of memory, physical activity will increase blood circulation, thereby helping to improve and maintain memory. Exercise provides more oxygen to the brain and allows the body an opportunity to cleanse itself of accumulated toxins, through perspiration. If your loved one is mobile, the easiest forms of exercise would include: walking, cycling, swimming, aerobics, and light gym workouts, such as treadmills and stationary bicycles. If this is not possible, there are exercises that can be done in a bed or on a chair. These exercises include: chair yoga, band exercises, and assisted stretching such as lifting arms and legs.

Did you know that it is more beneficial to walk outside as opposed to walking on a treadmill indoors? The Japanese believe that the practice of Shinrin Yoku, also known as forest bathing, is good for both physical and mental well-being. Shinrin Yoku can improve mood, lower heart rate and blood pressure, reduce the production of stress hormones, boost the immune system, and accelerate recovery from illness. Forest bathing is the conscious and contemplative practice of walking in the woods, taking in everything with all of one's senses. The sounds, the atmosphere, the smells, the temperature, and the beautiful, calming sights are all parts of the natural beauty your senses will delight in.

If your loved one is averse to traditional exercise, there are activities they can do that will still provide all the benefits associated with traditional exercise. Consider tai chi, yoga, dancing, gardening, or simply helping around the house with light or manufactured housework.

In this chapter, we reviewed a comprehensive list of holistic therapies and alternative care methods that show how Western and Eastern therapies can be used simultaneously to treat your loved one.

The holistic treatments we discussed are not only meant to alleviate the symptoms of the disease, but also to promote an overall sense of wellness, by taking care of physical, emotional, mental, and spiritual needs, which is done by treating the body as a whole, rather than just treating the symptoms.

Even though none of these treatments reverse or stop the progression of dementia, they do ensure that your loved one's life will have a higher quality. These treatments also attempt to provide your loved one with a sense of purpose and achievement, so that they can spend the remainder of their days with boosted morale and higher self-esteem.

I am sure you join me in wishing to improve the quality of life of your loved one, to the greatest extent possible, as we both want them to live the best possible version of their life.

Chapter 15
The Criticality of Self-Care for Dementia Caregivers

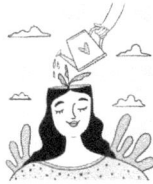

We have established how rewarding and fruitful caring for your loved one can be. Caregiving is an opportunity to spend quality time with your loved one during the final chapter of their life. However, what is equally important to understand, is that prolonged caregiving can be extremely overwhelming and exhausting. In addition, you will be faced with many challenges that can cause stress, and if not addressed, the emotional impact experienced will most assuredly take a toll on your mental and physical health, as well as, your state of mind. This can impact your personal relationships and ultimately lead to caregiver burnout.

Burnout is a state characterized by physical, emotional, and mental exhaustion. If and when you reach this point, both you and your loved one are sure to suffer. This is why, as I emphasized earlier, taking care of yourself and putting yourself first, is not a luxury; rather, it is an absolute necessity.

Recognizing symptoms early on can reduce and hopefully help you to avoid burnout. It is instrumental to understand what these symptoms look like because burnout doesn't happen in a single day, but over time when unchecked.

First, I will help you to recognize the various signs of caregiver stress, with the hope that we can stop this occurrence from taking place to begin with. Then, we'll look at the signs of caregiver burnout, so that we can stop it in its tracks, if it should arise.

Signs of Prolonged Caregiver Stress

If you have been taking care of your loved one for a prolonged period of time (more than a year), then you may have experienced some of these symptoms, especially if you're the primary (or only) caregiver for your loved one.

- Difficulty concentrating on everyday tasks
- Neglecting your personal responsibilities
- Reducing or eliminating activities and favorite hobbies
- Feeling signs of resentment
- Lethargy leading to feelings of defeat
- Difficulty both in falling and staying asleep
- Dealing with morbidity - anxiety, irritability, depression, stress, hopelessness, sadness, etc.
- Substance abuse - increased drinking, smoking, etc.
- Emotional eating - junk food
- Overreacting to insignificant issues
- Neglecting signs of potential health issues or allowing existing health problems to go unchecked, such as canceling or postponing doctor appointments

- Isolating yourself from friends and family

Signs of Caregiver Burnout

When the aforementioned symptoms are not addressed, they can escalate into caregiver burnout and you should be aware of the following signs:

- Feelings of aloneness, helplessness, hopelessness, which make it difficult to see the light at the end of the tunnel.
- A significant change in your energy level, regardless of what you do, including taking a nap and or taking a break; you feel drained and are unable to spark your prior energy level.
- Your immune system shows signs of decline. You find yourself catching every cold and bout of flu that is going around.
- Caregiving has enveloped every aspect of your life and you no longer feel satisfaction in your role as a caregiver.
- Relaxation has become difficult at best, even after you have had relief.
- You have become resigned and are neglecting your own personal needs because you are too busy caring for the needs of your loved one. It can get to the point, that your needs are now an afterthought.
- You have become impatient and irritable caring for your loved one.

Unfortunately, these signs are prevalent among caregivers. As the primary caregiver, it is necessary for you to understand that the long-term mental and physical consequences of burnout and stress can severely impact your own health, and can ultimately prevent you from being able to care for your loved one. Whether you have taken on the responsibility of your loved one due to an overwhelming sense of responsibility, guilt, obligation, denial, or just out of love, it is clear that you have elected to become your loved one's primary caregiver - so let's make sure you can do it, and do it well!

Strategies that You Can Utilize to Nip Stress in the Bud and Prevent it From Evolving into Full-blown Burnout

Emotional Self-Care

Much of the stress and burnout experienced is a result of a lack of emotional self-care, specifically when dealing with negative situations. If this is your first time as a caregiver, you are bound to be entering uncharted territory. This can lead to feelings of confusion and helplessness, as you may be unsure of how to handle these uniquely stressful situations. Understanding how to deal with these various forms of situations, can assist you when confronting these emotional challenges.

Forgive Yourself

You may not have all the answers, and things are not always going to go the way you plan or expect them to go. This rings truer when you are the caregiver for a person with dementia because it is not only a degenerative neurological disease, which over time, can radically alter the personality of your loved one, but it can turn your loved one into someone who is no longer the person you knew and loved - that's what makes it hurt so much and makes it so hard to deal with. The hands that once hugged you and made everything better, can now lash out to scratch, slap, or push you away. They may show signs of irritation, refuse to cooperate, and even become verbally abusive.

Acceptance and having an understanding of the situation and what's to come, is extremely important, because unfortunately, as the disease progresses, things are going to get worse, not better. Being asked the same question dozens of times and forgetting what is happening or who people are, is usually the first indication of decline. It is important that you understand this can and usually does exacerbate to the point that they no longer know who you are. This is one of the most difficult experiences you might have to endure as the primary caregiver for your loved one. All of these factors can contribute to your feelings of impatience, frustration, anger, resentment, sadness and loss. Do not feel that this is a reflection of the care you are giving. You are NOT a bad person. You are a wonderful human being. Caring for your loved one with dementia, is one of the most generous demonstrations of love 💕. Give yourself a hug. Extend kindness, forgiveness, and leniency toward the person who needs and deserves it the most - YOU. You are earning your wings day by day. Clearly, you are a special angel 😇 sent from heaven.

Have a Flexible Daily Plan

When dealing with dementia, no one can predict how the day will go, so don't set yourself up for failure by planning your day with unrealistic expectations. It is important to go with the flow and not worry about keeping to a rigid schedule; rather, adapt to the situation as needed and be willing and able to act accordingly. Every day (sometimes every hour), you will discover that your loved one's symptoms can vary significantly and they can become extremely difficult to deal with, while other days, they can seem to be in good humor. With a balanced and flexible approach to each day, you can avoid feelings of disappointment and frustration, so that if things do turn for the worse, you will be better prepared and better able to cope. Regardless, as the caregiver, you will do best embarking on this journey with an open mind. Although you might begin this endeavor with the mindset of caring for your loved one independently and feel that you will not require professional caregiving assistance, or a specialized dementia care facility, there may come a time when that is no longer possible - even if you do everything by the book, things may not always go as you had expected, or be in your control.

Cherish Those Moments of Connection (for they are a gift)

There may be times during your caregiving journey, when it will seem like your loved one has reverted to their old self - even if it's just for a bit of time. These moments are nothing short of a gift, allowing you to reconnect with your loved one, as in days of old. Honor and enjoy these moments! Talk, share, and just enjoy this special time together.

Another meaningful activity that you can do with your loved one, especially if they're in the earlier stage of dementia, is to take pictures, videos, write letters, and take part in activities. Later, all of these pictures, videos, and letters will become wonderful memories for when things get more difficult and, ultimately, when they are no longer with you.

When Someone Offers Help (say YES - without hesitation)

When a friend or family member offers to step in to provide you some relief, just say yes. It will allow that person an opportunity to feel involved and spend time with your (their) loved one and will also provide an opportunity for your loved one to have social interactions. Most importantly, it will also provide you with much-needed time you need, to take a break or simply relax.

We've already looked at other aspects related to emotional care, which have included: seeking a caregiver support group, arranging for social time, equipping yourself with information and knowledge so that you can anticipate what's going to happen, and creating a routine with your loved one that streamlines both your days. All of these care elements can help to avert burnout or the build-up of long-term stress that contributes to burnout.

Empower Yourself as a Caregiver - Think Positively and Practice Gratitude

Two of the major contributors of burnout are feelings of helplessness and lack of power, in the face of this disease, that's slowly taking your loved one from you. It is all too easy to fall into the trap of feeling helpless, especially if you never expected to be thrust into this role. What makes matters even worse, is the realization that there is nothing you or anyone else can do, to cure or reverse this disease.

You need to remember - you are not powerless. Repeat that again and again until you believe it - you are not powerless. Although you will be unable to revert your loved one to their pre-dementia self and you may not have the financial wherewithal, physical assistance, or time you need to better care for yourself, you can increase your hope, happiness, acceptance, and optimism. This will make all the difference in terms of gaining power.

Dwelling upon things you cannot change, expending your mental energy, trying to reason with the unfairness of this disease, and continually struggling with the situation that you are in, will not add any benefit, nor will it improve your situation. Rather than focus your time on negative thoughts, do your best to practice acceptance. This will enable you to avoid falling into the emotional trap of feeling sorry for yourself and your loved one, and with time and practice, you will begin to replace blame with understanding and gratitude. All of your energy should be channeled into taking pragmatic and practical steps toward making your loved one's life better, which will occur through empathetic caregiving. Empower yourself by focusing on all the positive reasons which lead you to the decision to be the caregiver for your loved one. Although reasons may vary, you have come to the decision to step up and take on this Herculean role. Maybe your decision was based on an opportunity to repay your loved one for all the years they loved and took care of you, or perhaps your decision was based on the values you embody, such as wanting to set an example for your children - family comes first. Or, it might have been to keep the promise you made to your loved one and want to keep. Remembering why you made this decision in the first place, will serve to strengthen your motivation to sustain yourself through these hard times.

While there are positive and negative aspects related to everything in life, choosing to focus on the positive aspects (the silver lining), such as looking at how caregiving has improved your own life by making you strong enough to rise to this challenge, or how it has brought you closer to your loved one - optimism and gratitude will help empower you.

Let's talk about gratitude. When you're in the thrusts of caregiving and can foresee the downhill struggle of your journey, things can get pessimistic and the world can seem dark. Although it's human nature to dwell on negative aspects, it is much healthier to focus on all and any positive aspects and remain hopeful. Cultivating gratitude in your life is both healthy and a beneficial means to stay grounded and happy.

As challenging and painful as the disease and its progression are to live with and as disheartening as it is to see your loved one in this condition, there's still reason to be grateful. Gratitude is not about ignoring bad things, rather it's about looking past those things and still being able to recognize all of the good things still going on in your life, that deserve appreciation.

You should be grateful that you're here and have the ability to care for your loved one in their time of need. Setting aside a few minutes every day, to actively reflect upon all the reasons you have to be grateful, and writing them down, in a gratitude journal, has been known to improve mental and physical health. Gratitude causes physiological changes in your body that initiate the parasympathetic nervous system. This is the part of your mind that helps you rest and digest. Gratitude helps lower blood pressure and heart rate and improves breathing, which is germain in achieving overall relaxation.

I believe a gratitude journal to be such an important tool in helping you achieve this goal, that I have provided a journal for you to use for this purpose.

If you are reading the ebook, click this link: https://bit.ly/3MNPzhm, or if you are reading the print version, scan the QR code below. I strongly suggest you take advantage of this tool.

Another important element of empowering yourself, revolves around appreciation. Make sure you receive the appreciation that you not only deserve, but need. You can achieve this in a variety of ways.

Supportive friends and family members can show their appreciation by acknowledging your hard work and offering you positive reinforcement. Don't forget to ask, for what you need. You can provide this to yourself, in the form of validation. You should applaud and acknowledge yourself for everything you've done and continue to do. Appreciation can also be obtained through a mental exercise. Imagine how much your loved one would appreciate all you are doing and all your efforts if they were healthy of mind and were able to respond and thank you for all you are doing for them during this time.

Focus on all the factors that are in your control, rather than those you have no control over. It is a given - problems will arise. It is how you face these problems that empower you.

Retain Your Individuality - Do Things That Bring You Joy

Most importantly, do not let caregiving become an all-consuming factor in your life. Be sure to stay in touch with friends and family; this includes making time for your own family (husband, children, grandchildren, etc.). Continue to participate in your favorite hobbies when possible and do your best, in some manner, to manage your career, if applicable. These are just some of the controllable variables, that will help you to feel empowered in the face of caregiving challenges.

Two musts: retain your individuality and your identity. Make sure you never lose yourself in your caregiving journey.

Maintaining Your Mental and Physical Health as a Caregiver

I have a personal story to share with you. When my sister and I were little, my mother would tell us, "On this earth, god has masterfully given us bodies to use as our vehicles to navigate the world, and we each get only one. It is up to each of us, to nourish and care for our vehicle to ensure its health, well-being, and longevity." She used this analogy by likening our bodies to a car. "You can have the best, most expensive car, but if you don't care for it properly, providing it the maintenance and fuel it needs, it won't run reliably; it can break down, and it won't last."

Life can be stressful, even under the best of conditions; however, caregiving adds yet another dimension of stress to our lives. Do not add to that stress by neglecting your health. Many health problems are both treatable and sometimes even avoidable - some can even be self-perpetuated. You should always keep your health at the forefront; however, while being a caregiver, it is of the utmost importance.

Get Regular Exercise

Exercise gets you out of your head and swaps cortisol (the primary stress hormone) with a healthy helping of dopamine and serotonin, which are integral chemicals that our body utilizes to elevate mood.

Quite often, when time is a factor, people will sacrifice their own time for that of their loved ones. Time at the gym or other forms of physical exercise, should not be one of those to sacrifice. This is one of the more important acts of self-care to maintain, especially as a caregiver. Whether you were playing a sport regularly or hitting a yoga class, if you feel that due to your caregiving responsibilities, you no longer have the time to do so, rearrange your day to make time for some form of physical exercise. An added bonus would be, if you could include your loved one, as both you and your loved one should get a daily dose of physical activity. To maintain your health, you have to make time in your day—if not hours, then minutes. Set aside whatever available time you can to walk, run, swim, cycle, do calisthenics, or even set up a home gym, if possible, so that you can continue to have the ability to maintain moderate-to-vigorous physical exercise in your life. There are really no excuses. If you literally cannot find any time in a given day, you can sprinkle them in by: dancing while you are cooking, doing leg lifts while you are washing the dishes, choosing the stairs over taking the elevator, putting ankle weights on, while you are vacuuming the carpet - the options are endless.

All of these activities will be instrumental in helping you retain your physical strength, improve your stamina, reduce stress, maintain your weight, regulate your blood pressure and cholesterol, and, it may even get you out of the house and away from caregiving, if only for a while. Even just sprinkling in some of those tips I mentioned, can ground you and relieve stress while replenishing and rejuvenating your body.

Remember, this can also be an opportunity for both you and your loved one to share time and be together by: taking a walk or wheeling your loved one outside, yoga, tai chi, putting on music that your loved one likes and dancing or moving to the music. Any of these activities can serve as a great bonding experience and has been proven to be beneficial both mentally and physically.

Look Out For Depression and Other Signs of Psychological Morbidity

Psychological morbidity can sneak up on you as a caregiver, especially when you're undergoing stress and anxiety. Depression can be exhibited in the form of apathy, tiredness, hopelessness, a lack of energy to do the things that you need or want to do, reduced or lack of interest in activities you once enjoyed, social isolation, and in its worse form, can lead to suicidal ideation. If you're experiencing any of these signs, you must get in touch with a mental health care professional. Depression is a manageable problem. With therapies like psychotherapy, talk therapy, and medication, depression and its symptoms can be addressed and mitigated.

Don't Forget About Your Own Doctor's Appointments

Understandably, the increased visits to the doctor with your loved one and the time you are putting into caregiving, can result in your foregoing your own health and visits to the doctor. Doing this can have very serious consequences. If you fall ill, and don't take the proper and necessary care of yourself, you can become so sick that you will be incapable of taking care of your loved one. Reminder Alert - don't forget to make appointments for your annual check-ups and other doctor visits, including labwork and preventative screenings. If something precludes you from keeping any of your appointment(s), make sure you make an alternate appointment ASAP and do not leave it as an open item on your to-do list. If you feel unhealthy or your body is giving you any abnormal symptoms, have yourself checked out as quickly as you can.

Eat Healthy

When taking care of a loved one with dementia, it is quite common to put your own needs in last place. Resorting to shortcuts when it comes to your needs, is not the answer. For instance, if you're running short on time and are feeling hungry, it might make sense to grab a quick bite at McDonald's, so that you don't have to go home and take the time to prepare a meal for yourself. After all, that time could go towards taking care of your loved one. But when such shortcuts compound, they can take a toll on your health, especially when it comes to your diet. A healthy diet, even if it means taking more time to prepare, will ensure you have more energy, will preserve your health, and can prevent any health problems associated with nutrition. As we discussed in previous chapters, a healthy diet, is especially necessary for your loved one, as diets high in sugar can be the cause of behavioral issues, increase cognitive decline, and exacerbate comorbidities.

Foods with healthy fats, such as olive oil, nuts, and fish are recommended, as are fresh fruits, veggies, and lean protein. Unlike caffeine and sugary foods, which only provide a short boost of energy, these healthier choices will fuel the body with long-term, steady energy.

In need of additional sources of energy, caregivers can begin to rely upon copious amounts of coffee, energy drinks, and cigarettes to satisfy this need. This is a trap you want to avoid. Although caffeine and nicotine can give you a boost of energy in the short term, dependence on these chemicals can become extremely harmful to your health, especially if you're indulging on a regular basis. Let's not forget, that smoking in and of itself is clearly, extremely toxic and is known to be a cause of lung disease and cancer, among other health issues - so don't smoke, and if you do - stop.

Reduce Stress

Relaxation techniques are underrated, criminally so, in my opinion. Yoga, meditation, tai chi, deep breathing exercises, muscle relaxation, and mindfulness are some relaxation techniques that allow you to feel more centered, reduce your stress levels, and boost your feelings of well-being and joy.

They can also help you focus on what's important so that you can let go of everything that's just holding you down.

If you take one thing away from this book, it is that self-care for you, the caregiver, is critical. Now that you are aware of the signs of caregiver stress and burnout, be mindful of them. Take breaks and ask for help when needed. Empower yourself as a caregiver and make your health a priority through regular exercise, healthy eating habits, and different forms and techniques for relaxation.

Chapter 16
Dealing With Family

The two major challenges that you, as the primary caregiver, will face when dealing with you and your loved one's family include:

- Coming to terms with the diagnosis
- Exploring and, when necessary, resolving conflicts with regard to the care of your loved one, and the associated responsibilities and decision-making that are necessary as the disease progresses

Coming to Terms with the Diagnosis

Just as you and your loved one will have to adjust to your new normal post-diagnosis life, so too will your family and friends. Although dementia will have a great impact on every aspect of your life, the most common feelings and emotions faced by your loved one and family members will be that of guilt, grief, loss, anger, sadness, and denial.

Tips to Help Comfort Family - Recognizing the Dynamics

A spouse, children and grandchildren, immediate and extended family members, and friends will all be affected and the complexities and nuances of each will require varying levels of sensitivity.

Spouse

If you are the primary caregiver, as well as the spouse of your loved one with dementia, you will need support coming to terms with the diagnosis and preliminary decisions. You can be overwhelmed by initial emotions resulting from your sense of loss, fears of loneliness, and guilt.

This is the time to be inclusive, do not isolate yourself or try to go this alone. The expression "it takes a village" was never more true. Just as you have assembled a team of healthcare professionals (discussed in prior chapters), it is time to assemble your support system and gather as much knowledge as you can, because knowledge will give you power. Be open to support from all avenues, as you never know where and from whom this knowledge will be derived.

Seeking various groups and activities with people in your area (or even online) can be instrumental in helping both you and your loved one, as other people who have gone through or are going through this life-changing challenge will be able to provide much-needed guidance and understanding. Together, you can attend early-stage caregiver support groups and connect with others who are going through a similar situation. Knowing that there are others sharing your fears and concerns can be instrumental in coming to terms and hopefully, will give you much-needed support during this time.

Continued participation in favorite activities can be both enjoyable, as well as, provide an opportunity to include your loved one in areas that can both exercise their brain, as well as, help to keep them socially engaged, for as long as possible. This might be the last opportunity you will have to fulfill any open items on their bucket list. Be sure to allow important people in their lives the opportunity to visit and spend time. Be sure to create lasting memories and stories that you will be happy to have to pass down from generation to generation.

Children and Grandchildren

If there are young children or grandchildren in the household, including them in their loved one's care will be essential in determining their acceptance and thwarting those feelings associated with fear and distress. Depending upon their age and ability to comprehend the disease, you should explain how the disease will affect and change their loved one, at a level appropriate to their understanding. As the primary caregiver, you should consider many of the various ways you can include them, so that they can spend time and support their loved one. If you feel the situation is creating any adverse feelings, consider having them see a counselor who specializes in families dealing with such illnesses.

Notifying your children's school would be advisable, so that any change in behavior can be more easily understood and addressed. It is important to provide a positive atmosphere, as the last thing you would want is a home environment filled with depression and sadness. Including your loved one and children in light-hearted, fun activities would be beneficial to everyone. Remember that laughter has a healing effect and makes everyone happier. As an aside, you should note that children tend to take their cues from their parents and older siblings, so, if you treat your loved one with love and respect and shelter them from feelings of fear and agitation - that behavior will most likely be mimicked by them. One day, when you are older and possibly in need of assistance, you will thank yourself, when your children and/or grandchildren are there to support your needs and will do so in a loving, caring manner, for which you set the example. Creating a "normal environment" will yield your children feeling that things are normal - just different.

Friends and Extended Family

Your loved one's friends, extended family, co-workers, and neighbors will not necessarily understand what is going on. Even if they surmise what is happening, they might be conflicted as to what they should do or say. Some may maintain their distance and, over time, lose touch. Others may be uncomfortable approaching the subject and wait for you to reach out. Therefore, my suggestion is to be inclusive and share the diagnosis early on by letting them know that their love is appreciated and welcome.

Remember, "it takes a village." If they offer their assistance during this time, be gracious and let them know how they can help and support you and your loved one. This opportunity will not only be advantageous to you and your loved one, but will also give them a way to feel included and may be helpful to them in processing their own feelings of loss and grief.

Conflict Resolution

In some cases, the inability to adjust can cause conflicts to ensue between family members. To understand why these conflicts arise in the first place, we have to keep in mind that the news of the diagnosis sparks feelings of uncertainty, grief, loss, anger, guilt, sadness, and sacrifice. These emotions will affect the quality of life of your loved one, as well as their relatives and friends.

As secondary caregivers, family members and friends can be conflicted by their feelings associated with their role. They might graciously volunteer their time and truly want to help, without realizing how it may intrude on their time and potentially require them to reprioritize their existing relationships, lifestyle, and activities. Communication is key. As the primary caregiver, you should be clear and encourage an honest, open dialogue so that each person assisting you with the care of your loved one understands that **anything** they can do is greatly appreciated and no effort is too small. It is important that they feel good about what they do and not guilty about what they cannot do. And, if done without resentment but rather empathy and love, the gift will be better received and have the best result.

Dementia can be an extremely isolating disease. Suddenly, the person who everyone relied upon, has a disease that will deteriorate their mind and body. You are losing this person you know and love, slowly over time. As mentioned above, "it takes a village"- find your village.

After the diagnosis, some family members and friends will prefer to have nothing to do with the process. There could be a number of reasons for them opting out. Counterintuitive as it may seem, it is okay. Let them be. Caregiving is a huge responsibility and it should be a conscious one. It shouldn't be forced upon someone, especially if they're not willing or able to be there for their (your) loved one. There are many reasons that can cause conflict during this time. Some family members might try to exploit the situation in an emotional, financial, or legal way. This is not a harmless behavior, and you should consult an attorney to understand what laws are available to protect your loved one from being exploited by family members.

Conflict may also arise as a result of guilt. Family members and friends may be torn, wondering if they're doing enough for your (their) loved one, or shirking their responsibilities. Frustration also contributes to conflict, especially as it revolves around your (their) loved one's inability to respond as they would have in the past. Empathy can go a long way here, especially when resolving conflicts between family members. Opening lines of empathetic communication, where each family member has an opportunity to listen and be heard, can not only resolve a conflict but also bring to light the varying opinions available to each family member. Opinions might also spark arguments regarding finances, caregiving decisions, and end-of-life planning. Even if your loved one has already designated a power of attorney, these discussions may still come into play, but know that the ultimate decision is that of the person designated as the power of attorney.

These are all very complex issues that require constant communication and discussion where everyone has an opportunity to share their opinions without blaming each other, attacking each other, and hurting each other's sentiments. That's where empathy comes in. If you keep in mind that your family members are going through the same thing that you are and possibly are processing it differently, this understanding will help to diminish many conflicts and potentially make those still existing, easier to resolve.

Delegate caregiving responsibilities to different family members and friends (when possible), so that no one person is overburdened with all responsibilities and everyone has a reasonable number of tasks delegated to them. This can help to avoid potential conflicts. Another source of conflict can come into play when family members feel they are being kept out of the loop. This can cause resentment by feelings associated with dejection and/or exclusion. Keeping an open line of communication with the entire family through regular messaging, weekly or monthly conference calls, or regular meetings will keep everyone up-to-date and can keep everyone abreast of what is happening, which will provide a sense of involvement in the caregiving process.

Playing the blame game is not uncommon for some when hearing this diagnosis. As irrational as it may seem, it is natural to look for a cause and assign blame to that cause.

With so many conflicting emotions and feelings of fear and confusion, it is not uncommon to point fingers and place blame on each other for the disease. These feelings usually come into play, when in the denial stage of this disease. When struggling to come to terms with the diagnosis, it is easy to lash out at others, which is a natural defense mechanism. Remember, knowledge is power, and hopefully, as the primary caregiver, you have armed yourself with enough knowledge on the disease so that you are able to communicate, grieve, and help others have a better understanding of what is happening. Do your best to convey that this is a terrible disease, but there are no "bad guys" to blame in this narrative. Try to encourage them to research information, so that they can have a better understanding and come to the realization that you are all on the same team. Remind them that you are all a TEAM - together, everyone achieves more. This would be a perfect time to suggest they retain a copy of this book or order it for them as a gift!

If necessary, family members can seek assistance from a third party, such as a counselor, religious leader, or therapist. Sometimes, an outside, objective perspective can help in working through conflicts.

Although these tips and strategies should prove helpful, coming to terms with accepting the diagnosis is very difficult for family members and loved ones to endure. Having a support system and coming together during this difficult time should be helpful to each team member. Remember to avoid conflicts amongst yourselves, at any cost. This painful time in your life will become more bearable when you, your family members, and loved ones have each other to lean on.

My hope, is that through the strategies and tips provided in this chapter, you and your family will have the framework of support, information, and guidance, to utilize and help each other avoid conflicts, during this difficult time.

Afterword

When I decided to write this book, I felt compelled to offer assistance to potential caregivers dealing with a loved one diagnosed with dementia. My paternal grandmother and both her daughters, my aunts, were victims of this disease. As a pharmacist, I have developed specialized skills in elder care, which has added to my medical perspective, relating to dementia. I wrote this book for you, the caregiver, with the hope you would benefit from the information and stories encompassed within the sixteen chapters of this book. My family and I would have greatly benefited by having such a book, to use as a resource, and hope that the stories, information, and tips encompassed within this book, prove to be of great value to you, the caregiver, your loved one, and your family and friends. It's my way of giving back and honoring my loved ones.

I truly hope that I have accomplished my goal, and after having read this book, you have a better understanding of what is entailed in becoming a caregiver, the challenges that await you, and the strategies and tips you can implement to meet these obstacles head-on. I have done my best to illustrate the various stages of dementia, revealing the fulfilling journey and rewards associated with caring for your loved one with dementia, without sugarcoating the difficult journey you are about to embark on. Without a doubt, becoming a caregiver for your loved one is the most selfless responsibility you can take on. It is one of the highest forms of expressing your love, while enabling your loved one to retain the best possible quality of life, and preserving your loved one's dignity.

Writing this book and having readers such as yourself join me on your path is a humbling experience and I am very grateful to you for utilizing the resources I have provided. Having personally walked the walk myself, I genuinely know how difficult a decision it is to become a caregiver for your loved one with dementia. It is with sincere emotional understanding that I wrote each word in this book, hoping to both reach and educate you on your huge undertaking. Please utilize the tips, strategies, and advice I share, where applicable, so that you can provide your loved one with the best care possible, while avoiding common traps that first-time caregivers can so easily fall into.

I want to thank you for your time (which I know is sparse) in reading this book. I hope and wish you the strength, fortitude, and courage while sharing this challenging time with your loved one.

Always here to help,

Alison Blaire

Thank You

I would like to take this opportunity to extend my sincerest gratitude to you for taking the time to read my book. As an author, there is no greater joy than knowing that your words have reached and touched someone's heart. I hope my book has provided valuable insights, lessons, and comfort in your journey of caring for your loved one with dementia.

Your support means the world to me, and I am grateful for each and every one of you. Lastly, I would like to kindly ask for your help in leaving a review on Amazon.

By sharing your thoughts and experiences, you can help others in need of this important resource. Your review also allows me to hear about your journey and how my book has impacted your life. Thank you once again for choosing to read my book.
To leave a review, go to this link: http://amazon.com/review/create-review?&asin=B0CP9Z4B2Z

or scan the QR code below

Free Gift

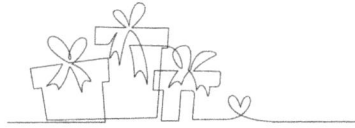

I am beyond grateful for your purchase of my book. To express my gratitude, I would like to gift you with a FREE activity book filled with mazes and word searches specifically designed to entertain and improve cognitive function. It's the perfect activity for you and your loved one to enjoy together! Simply use this **link: https://bit.ly/3Q81wAk** or scan the QR code below to access your free download.

Resources

Alzheimer's Association. (n.d.). What is dementia? [Brochure]. https://www.alz.org/alzheimers-dementia/what-is-dementia

National Institute on Aging. (2022, May 17). What is dementia? https://www.nia.nih.gov/health/what-is-dementia

Mayo Clinic. (2021, November 10). Diagnosis & treatment. Mayo Foundation for Medical Education and Research. https://www.mayoclinic.org/diseases-conditions/dementia/diagnosis-treatment/drc-20352019#:~:text=The%20following%20are%20used%20to,and%20galantamine%20(Razadyne%20ER)

Better Health Channel. (2019, August). Dementia - behavior changes. Victorian Government. https://www.betterhealth.vic.gov.au/health/conditionsandtreatments/dementia-behaviourchanges#:~:text=This%20is%20known%20as%20sundowning,t%20real%2C%20especially%20at%20night

Stanford Health Care. (n.d.). Causes of dementia. https://stanfordhealthcare.org/medical-conditions/brain-and-nerves/dementia/causes.html

National Institute on Aging. (2022, May 17). What happens to the brain in Alzheimer's disease? https://www.nia.nih.gov/health/what-happens-brain-alzheimers-disease

Alzheimer's Association. (n.d.). Types of dementia. https://www.alz.org/alzheimers-dementia/what-is-dementia/types-of-dementia

A Place for Mom. (n.d.). Dementia stages: How to recognize and identify the stages of dementia. https://www.aplaceformom.com/caregiver-resources/articles/dementia-stages

Mayo Clinic. (2021, November 10). Diagnosis & treatment. Mayo Foundation for Medical Education and Research. https://www.mayoclinic.org/diseases-conditions/dementia/diagnosis-treatment/drc-20352019

WebMD. (n.d.). Dementia Treatment Overview. https://www.webmd.com/alzheimers/dementia-treatments-overview

Alzheimer's Association. (n.d.). Building a Care Team. https://www.alz.org/help-support/i-have-alz/plan-for-your-future/building_a_care_team

Everyday Health. (n.d.). Doctors for Alzheimer's Disease: Who Should Be on Your Healthcare Team? https://www.everydayhealth.com/alzheimers-disease/doctors-for-alzheimers-disease-who-should-be-on-your-healthcare-team/

HelpGuide.org. (n.d.). Alzheimer's and Dementia Caregiving: How to Deal with Aggression and Other Behavioral Problems.

https://www.helpguide.org/articles/alzheimers-dementia-aging/alzheimers-behavior-management.htm

Alzheimer's Association. (n.d.). In-Home Care. https://www.alz.org/help-support/caregiving/care-options/in-home-care

Brookdale Senior Living. (n.d.). What is Memory Care? https://www.brookdale.com/en/our-services/memory-care/what-is-memory-care.html#: ~:text=Memory%20-care%20is%20a%20kind, the%20health%20of%20the%20residents

Five Star Senior Living. (n.d.). What Is the Difference Between Assisted Living and Nursing Homes? https://www.fivestarseniorliving.com/blog/what-is-the-difference-between-assisted-living-and-nursing-homes#:~:text=In%20assist-ed%20living%2C%20residents%20may,the%20-clock%20care%20and%20monitoring

A Place for Mom. (n.d.). Assisted Living vs. Memory Care. https://www.aplaceformom.com/caregiver-resources/articles/assisted-living-vs-memory-care

Alzheimer's Association. (n.d.). Hospice Care. https://www.alz.org/help-support/caregiving/care-options/hospice-care#:

~:text=Hospice%20care%20focuses%20on%20comfort,oth-er%20dementias%20and%20their%20families

HelpGuide.org. (n.d.). Tips for Alzheimer's Caregivers. https://www.helpguide.org/articles/alzheimers-dementia-aging/tips-for-alzheimers-caregivers.htm

Alzheimers.gov. (n.d.). Tips for Caregivers. https://www.alzheimers.gov/life-with-dementia/tips-caregivers

Alzheimer's Association. (n.d.). Stages and Behaviors. https://www.alz.org/help-support/caregiving/stages-behaviors

National Institute on Aging. (2022, May 17). Legal and Financial Planning for People with Alzheimer's. https://www.nia.nih.gov/health/legal-and-financial-planning-people-alzheimers

Alzheimer's Society. (n.d.). Legal and financial planning. https://www.alzheimers.org.uk/get-support/legal-financial

Alzheimer's Association. (n.d.). Financial and Legal Planning. https://www.alz.org/help-support/caregiving/financial-legal-planning

Alzheimer's Association. (n.d.). Plan for Your Future: Legal Planning. https://www.alz.org/help-support/i-have-alz/plan-for-your-future/legal_planning

Alzheimer's Association. (n.d.). Plan for Your Future: Financial Planning. https://www.alz.org/help-support/i-have-alz/plan-for-your-future/financial_planning

Alzheimer's Association. (n.d.). Management of Alzheimer's and Dementia Patients [Brochure]. https://www.alz.org/professionals/health-systems-medical-professionals/management

Alzheimer's Association. (n.d.). Medications for Memory [Brochure]. https://www.alz.org/alzheimers-dementia/treatments/medications-for-memory

Alzheimer's Association. (n.d.). Food and Eating [Brochure]. https://www.alz.org/help-support/caregiving/daily-care/food-eating#:

~:text=Offer%20vegetables%2C%20fruits%2C%20w-hole%20grains,and%20fatty%20cuts%20of%20meats

Alzheimer's Association. (n.d.). Reducing Stress [Brochure]. https://www.alz.org/help-support/i-have-alz/live-well/reducing-stress#:

~:text=Tips%20to%20reduce%20stress,-Identify%20sources%20of&text=Address%20the

%20triggers%20that%20are,for%20the%20posi-tive%20whenever%20possible

Dignity Health. (n.d.). What Is Holistic Health Care, Anyway? https://www.dignityhealth.org/articles/what-is-holistic-health-care-anyway#:~:text=Treating%20the%20Whole%20You,as-pect%20affects%20you%20in%20others

ComfortCare Homes. (n.d.). Holistic Dementia Treatment: The 4 Pillars of Success. https://comfortcarehomes.com/blog/80/holistic-dementia-treatment/#:

~:text=4%20Pillars%20of%20Holistic%20

Dementia,of%20treatment%

20to%20be%20successful

Neural Effects. (n.d.). Dementia Treatment at Home: Natural Ways to Help Your Loved One. https://neuraleffects.com/blog/dementia-treatment-at-home-natural/

Peprah, K. (2019, July 17). *Medical Cannabis for the Treatment of Dementia: A Review of Clinical Effectiveness and Guidelines*. NCBI Bookshelf. https://www.ncbi.nlm.nih.gov/books/NBK546328/#

Alzheimer Society of Canada. (n.d.). Alternative Treatments for Dementia. https://alzheimer.ca/en/about-dementia/how-can-i-treat-dementia/alternative-treatments-dementia

Choosing Therapy. (n.d.). Emotional Self-Care: What It Is and Why It Matters. https://www.choosingtherapy.com/emotional-self-care/

Verywell Mind. (2022, March 17). Stress and Burnout: Symptoms and Causes. https://www.verywellmind.com/stress-and-burnout-symptoms-and-causes-3144516

American Heart Association. (n.d.). Top 10 Caregiver Tips for Staying Healthy and Active. https://www.heart.org/en/health-topics/caregiver-support/top-10-caregiver-tips-for-staying-healthy-and-active

Verywell Mind. (2022, March 17). Stress and Burnout: Symptoms and Causes. https://www.verywellmind.com/stress-and-burnout-symptoms-and-causes-3144516

Alzheimer's Association. (2019, October 7). 10 Ways to Help a Family Living with Alzheimer's. https://www.alz.org/blog/alz/october-2019/10_ways_to_help_a_family_living_with_alzheimer_s

HelpGuide.org. (n.d.). Tips for Alzheimer's Caregivers. https://www.helpguide.org/articles/alzheimers-dementia-aging/tips-for-alzheimers-caregivers.htm

Family Caregiver Alliance. (n.d.). A Caregiver's Guide to Understanding Dementia Behaviors [Brochure]. https://www.caregiver.org/resource/caregivers-guide-understanding-dementia-behaviors/

Johns Hopkins Medicine. (n.d.). Facing Dementia in the Family [Brochure]. https://www.hopkinsmedicine.org/health/conditions-and-diseases/dementia/facing-dementia-in-the-family

Better Health Channel. (n.d.). Dementia - advice for families [Brochure]. https://www.betterhealth.vic.gov.au/health/conditionsandtreatments/dementia-advice-for-families

www.ingramcontent.com/pod-product-compliance
Lightning Source LLC
Chambersburg PA
CBHW032055020426
42335CB00011B/347